MW00889472

pregnancy care

With Ayurveda, Yoga & Acupressure.

Bhavisha Jhaveri

Note:

This book is not intended as a substitute for personal medical advice. The reader should consult a midwife or doctor in all matters relating to health and particularly in respect of any symptoms that may require diagnosis or medical attention. While the advice and information in this book is believed to be accurate and true at the time of going to press, neither the author nor publisher can accept any legal responsibility or liability for any errors or omissions that may be made.

First Edition : 2016

Second Edition : 2020

ISBN-: 978-1537476230

E-mail : bhavishajhaveri@gmail.com

Copyright © 2016 Bhavisha Jhaveri

All rights reserved.

No part of this publication may be reproduced, transmitted or stored in a retrieval system in any form or by any means, electronic, mechanical, photocopying, recording or otherwise, without the prior permission of the author.

Thanks a lot….

I thank God to direct me into the journey of writing this book, to give me strength, vision and adequate intelligence to understand the concept of ancient Ayurveda, Yoga and Acupressure and ability to put them in words.

I really thank my parents for their valuable support in the whole journey of writing this book.

I am very thankful to my supporting term to make this book refined and polished.

Supporting term…

Editorial Team: Hiral Jhaveri, Niyati Jhaveri, Shikha Patel,

Dhara Shah, Vidhi Parekh, Pragati Chandarana

Cover page and vector design: Tejash Gajjar

Model in the Book: Mrs. Dimple Shah and Master Chaitanya

From the Author

Pregnancy is a special time in a woman's life, a unique journey to a new and exciting future. Pregnancy is also a time of great physical, emotional and social change, a time to look to new responsibilities, to explore, to learn new things about one-self and happiness. It also involves lots of doubts and confusion.

This book will help to answer many of your questions. It is a mixture of three great natural therapies which combines Ayurveda, Yoga and Acupressure. This book speaks about more traditional aspects and lots of natural treatment for common problems.

It will guide you about preparation for pregnancy, physical and emotional changes experienced, care, monthly development and special diet during pregnancy. It includes exclusive section for pre and postnatal yoga, and excellent meditation techniques. A detailed coverage of acupressure therapy to solve most pre and postnatal problems. Description about labor process, breast feeding and many more...

Hope this book helps to solve your questions, anxiety and fears. Enjoy this once in a lifetime period and the future to come. I dedicate this book to all the mothers-to be, and wish them a prosperous and healthy unique journey.

What is the motive of the book?
Ayurveda says that the baby is combination of three phenomena i.e. 1) Its own destiny (past life karma) 2) The qualities and defects of its parents (sperm and ovum) 3) The treatment and care it receives during pregnancy. So it is indeed in the hands of parents, what kind of creation they want. We can work on final two options to have a physically, mentally and spiritually magnificent baby. This book aims to explore many colorful aspects and treatments to fulfill the entire journey.

Is the given information innovative?
No, the given information is not my own innovation. The knowledge shared have already been described by the great Ayurveda, ancient Yoga and traditional Acupressure. As an author I have tried to analyze, compact the views in a more approachable perspective.

Who are my target readers?
All beautiful ladies who are thinking to be charming mom, rather both parents who are ready to correct their own physical, mental and spiritual well being to conceive physically, mentally and spiritually divine baby.

Table of Contents

Preparing For Pregnancy

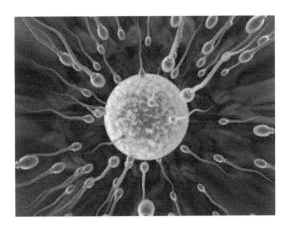

Pregnancy should be by choice, not by chance. Generally women do take very good care during pregnancy but there is seldom awareness about the importance of preparing for pregnancy as it is equally an important aspect.

According to Ayurveda child is a combination of three phenomena:

- Its own destiny (past life karma)
- The qualities and defects of its parents (sperm and ovum)
- The treatment and care it receives during pregnancy

We can work on last two options and in this chapter we will talk about the second last point which is 'the qualities and defects of its parents (sperm and ovum)' as the ultimate constitution of an individual is determined by the chromosomes of sperm and ovum and the health status of both the partners.

Eggs and sperms are the result of the deepest level of nutritional transformation. All that we eat and drink gets continually refined until it is transformed into the most vital essence, the potential of life, known as 'shukra' in Sanskrit. This is the seed of life. Ayurveda believes that if there are any obstructions in the body then the reproductive system becomes deficient and it is necessary to undergo rejuvenation for best production. Thus ideally pregnancy starts about six months before conception as both partners prepare themselves for the magical act of creation.

Knowledge of pregnancy is not only a science but also an art, and this is very well described by the great ancient Ayurveda.

In this book we have tried to cover all the topics related to pregnancy – from preparing for pregnancy, to the care of the mother and her baby, coupled with excellent remedies for some common illnesses the mother and the baby might experience and also solutions for all pre and post-natal care according to Ayurveda, Yoga and Acupressure.

In this first chapter we will talk about some interesting topics like the anatomy and physiology of the reproductive system, how menstrual cycle and pregnancy occurs, what is required for the best creation, and many more topics relating to how you can prepare yourself for pregnancy. So let's begin!

1.1   Anatomy and physiology of the reproductive system

It is vital to understand the reproductive system first. The main organs of the female reproductive system are vagina, cervix, uterus, fallopian tubes and ovaries, which can be seen below.

Vagina is like an external hole of the genitals. It is approximately 10 cm in length, and its other end connects to the cervix. It has various different functions, the most important one is to secrete a sticky mucus substance to prevent infection and lubricate itself so that sexual intercourse becomes easy and pain-free. It also expels menstrual blood and the fetus out, and lets the sperm enter.

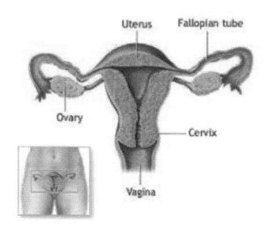

Female Reproductive System

The second part is the cervix, which is an opening or neck of the uterus. During pregnancy, the cervix remains closed, and its reopening is a sign of labor in progress. Interestingly, cervical tissues are not sensitive to touch, temperature or pain.

The third important part is the uterus, which is a hollow organ. It is approximately 5x8 cm (2x3.1 inches) in size and weigh 50-80 gm (1.7-2.8 ounces). Its walls are about 1.25 cm (0.50 inch) thick. The muscles of the uterus are greatly flexible and stretchable. It is an extraordinary organ and can expand 4 to 5 times more than its normal size and weigh up to 1 kg (2.2 pounds) during pregnancy, which gradually returns to its normal size and weight within 45 days of post-delivery. Its main role is to do with the production and expulsion of menstrual blood, planting the fertile seed, protection and nourishment of the fetus, development of the placenta and finally delivering the baby at the right time.

The fourth part is fallopian tubes, which extends out from both sides of the uterus. They are hollow, thin pipes of muscles, about 10 cm (4 inches) long, 1 cm (0.39 inches) wide with a diameter of about 1 cm (0.39 inches). Fallopian tubes are designed in the shape of half-open hibiscus flower and their main role is to catch the ovum from ovaries and lead it toward the uterus.

The last and key organ is the ovary. There are two of them, one on each side of the uterus, below a fallopian tube. Each ovary is about 3x2x1 cm (1.2x0.75x0.4 inches) in size. Each ovary releases one egg every alternate month, which means one ovary is active at any given time. Its main role is to produce a mature ovum, release it and to produce hormones.

How the menstrual cycle and pregnancy occurs

At the beginning of the cycle (first day of your period), an interesting process begins. A follicle-stimulating hormone (FSH) is produced by the pituitary gland in your brain, which is the main hormone for stimulating your ovaries to produce mature eggs. The FSH stimulates a number of follicles in your ovaries to develop and start producing the hormone estrogen. Your estrogen level is at its lowest on the first day of your period, but from then on, it starts to increase as the follicles grow.

Since a number of follicles begin to develop, normally one of them becomes dominant, and the egg matures within that enlarging follicle. At the same time, the increasing amount of estrogen in your body makes sure that the lining of your uterus is thickening with nutrients and blood. This happens so that if you get pregnant, the fertilized egg will have all the nutrients and support it needs for growing. High estrogen levels are also associated with the appearance of 'sperm-friendly' mucus (technically known as fertile cervical mucus). You may notice this as thin, slippery discharge that may be cloudy white. The advantage of this mucus is that sperm can swim more easily through it and can survive in it for several days.

The level of estrogen in your body continues to rise, eventually causing a rapid rise in luteinizing hormone, called the 'LH surge', which causes the dominant follicle to rupture and release its mature egg from its ovary into the fallopian tube. This process is known as ovulation. The egg (or ovum) has begun its first journey!

In general, this happens on the 12th or 14th day in the 28 day menstrual cycle, but it can vary cycle to cycle.

Once the egg is released, it moves along the fallopian tube towards the uterus (or womb). The egg can live for up to 24 hours, but sperm's survival is more variable, typically 3-5 days, so the days leading up to ovulation and the day of ovulation itself are the most fertile days and one is most likely to get pregnant during that time. As soon as you have ovulated, the follicle starts producing another hormone, progesterone, which causes further build-up of the lining of the womb in preparation for receiving a fertilized egg.

After ejaculation, sperm swims very quickly from the vagina into the cervix, through the uterus and into the fallopian tube towards the waiting egg. The egg helps the sperm by releasing chemicals attracting them towards itself. The race is on! Millions of sperms compete to penetrate the egg, out of which only one will succeed.

Once the egg has been fertilized, it tries to implant itself into the womb lining. This takes about a week after fertilization.

As soon as the fertilized egg has been implanted, your body starts producing the pregnancy hormone, human Chorionic Gonadotropin (hCG), which keeps the empty follicle actively produce the hormones – estrogen and progesterone. These hormones prevent the lining of the womb from being shed, until the placenta, which provides all the nutrients the embryo needs, is mature enough to maintain the pregnancy.

On the other hand, if the egg is not fertilized, the levels of estrogen and progesterone decreases. Without high levels of hormones, the thick womb lining that has been built up, starts to break down and your body sheds it. This marks the start of your period and beginning of your next menstrual cycle.

1.2   For a Healthy Reproductive System

According to Acharya Sushruta (an ancient Ayurvedic physician), "In the process of bringing about a healthy crop, it is essential that the season is appropriate, the soil is cured, the provision of water is optimum and the seed is of high quality. Similarly, for ideal conception, it is necessary that the season and occasion are suitable for the mother-to-be, her womb is free of all illnesses, the availability of nutrition for development of fetus is optimum, and the seed (i.e. sperm and ovum) is healthy and potent."

Then a natural question arises, "How healthy are my ovum, womb and whole reproductive system at present? Are they ready for conception?"

Ayurveda has given a beautiful answer to this question! It says that a healthy menstrual cycle indicates a healthy reproductive system.

But that begs the question too. How do I know if I have a healthy menstrual cycle? What are the characteristics of a healthy menstrual cycle?

And here is the answer. Ideally your period should:

- Take place every 28 days
- Last for 4-5 days
- Be free of any pain, discomfort and burning sensation
- Be odor free and leave stains on cotton cloth that are easily washable under running water
- Discharge blood of bright-bright red color
- Discharge blood that is not sticky and is free of clots
- Discharge approximately 40-80 gm (1.4-2.8 ounces) of blood

If all of these are true for you, you are lucky! You are having a perfectly healthy reproductive system that is ready for conception. But if these are not true for you, the good news is that Ayurveda suggests steps you can take to improve the situation. So first you refine your health, then plan for conception, whilst having the resource of a healthy system.

Let's now explore both of these situations to find out more about them – 1) You don't have a healthy reproductive system and 2) You do have a healthy reproductive system.

What If You Don't Have a Healthy Reproductive System?

One of the main reason for hormonal imbalances that harm reproductive systems is choosing wrong diet and lifestyle such as consumption of inappropriate food, unnecessary strain, stress, excess mental work, lack of physical workout, lack of proper rest etc leads to hormonal imbalance and finally results into poor reproductive system and poor menstrual cycle. For example, excess mental work, stress, staying awake till late night, excess consumption of junk food leads to imbalance in *vata dosha*. Excess consumption of very oily or spicy food, unnecessary strain and stress, lack of proper rest, etc. imbalances *pitta dosh*. Lack of exercise, excess consumption of sweet and high fat diet, sedentary lifestyle, etc. imbalances *kapha dosha*.

According to Ayurveda, imbalances in *vata, pitta*, and *kapha doshas* can lead to imbalance in the menstrual flow which can be identified by following symptoms:

Symptoms of imbalance in menstrual flow

Dosha imbalance	Menstrual imbalance
Vata dosha	Painful, scanty discharge; dark or blackish discharge
Pitta dosha	Excess bleeding, foul-smelling discharge, burning sensation
Kapha dosha	Sticky and mucoid discharge
All three dosha	Scanty, painful, foul-smelling discharge accompanied by clots

Measures to help these imbalances

- **Scanty/Painful Menstruation**
  Symptoms
  o   Delayed menstruation
  o   Reduced bleeding or short menstruation
  o   Painful menstruation
  o   Blood flowing in clots

  Causes
  o   Low hemoglobin level (anemia)
  o   Low calcium level
  o   Imbalance of vata dosha
  o   Excessive thinking or stress
  o   Thyroid dysfunction

  Treatment
  o   Food rich in hemoglobin should be consumed, such as dates, pomegranate, spinach, raagi (finger millet) etc.
  o   Food having abundant calcium should be consumed, such as milk, milk products, amla (Indian gooseberry), papaya, banana etc.
  o   Aloe Vera is highly beneficial. Medications such as Kumari Asav and Ashokarista etc, which are prepared from Aloe Vera works excellent.
  o   Abdominal massage (ideally with castor oil) and abdominal exercises such as cycling, crunches, leg raising, etc. are advantageous.
  o   Hot hip-bath during and 4-5 days prior to the period. This is very fruitful naturopathy treatment.
  o   Acupressure – Please refer to Chapter 5.

- **Excess Menstrual Discharge**

  Symptoms
  - Excessive bleeding
  - Long periods lasting 6 to 10 days
  - Very short period cycle of 15 to 21 days

  Causes
  - Imbalance of *pitta dosha*
  - Hot weather
  - Consumption of excess spicy food
  - Stress
  - Thyroid dysfunction
  - Tumor in uterus, tubes or ovaries

  Treatment
  - Avoid oily, spicy and fermented food
  - Drink Neem juice + Jeera (black cumin) every day for a week
  - Consume calcium, Vitamins C and K rich food
  - Eat *gulkand* (rose petals jam), soaked raisins, *mishri* (crystalized sugar), fennel seed, etc. to expel excess heat from the body
  - Acupressure – Please refer to Chapter 5.

- **Vaginal Discharge/White Discharge**

  Discharge of white, sticky or watery fluid is normal, only if it occurs 1-2 days prior to the onset of menstruation or at the time of ovulation. But a discharge at any other time is anomalous. It is advisable to seek attention for this, even if the quantity of discharge is negligible.

  Symptoms
  - Vaginal discharge
  - Weakness, dizziness, backache, leg pain, headache
  - Gas formation, lack of sound sleep, lack of appetite

  Causes
  - Constipation
  - Excess sexual activity
  - Excess physical work
  - Weak uterus
  - Excess heat in body

Treatment
- o   *Harde powder* (Terminalia chebula) works excellent
- o   Consumption of buttermilk in good quantity
- o   Consumption of *ashwagandha powder* (Withania somnifera) with milk
- o   Regular exercise and yoga
- o   Drinking rice water
- o   Acupressure – Please refer to Chapter 5.

- **Thyroid Dysfunction**

  Thyroid hormone imbalance is one of the major causes of anomalous period cycle. This imbalance comes from an unhealthy lifestyle, poor food habits, stress, and careless behavior during menstruation.

  Symptoms

  The symptoms can range from swelling of the body, to weight gain, to increase in blood pressure etc.

  Treatment
  - o   Yoga practices
  - o   Meditation to relieve stress
  - o   Acupressure – Please refer to Chapter 5.

This brief discussion on the symptoms and treatments of an unhealthy period cycle should give an idea one can apply to one's own situation. It is highly recommended to ensure healthy periods before planning for conception.

You can also visit a good Ayurvedic doctor (*Vaidya*), but let your periods be healthy for three consecutive cycles before you plan a baby.

You may have a question, why is it important to have healthy periods for three consecutive cycles?

The sole reason is the health and vitality of the baby! As we have already discussed that a child is a combination of three phenomena and through this, we are working on the second last option of the health of the ovum.

Now that we've had a brief understanding about what can be done to have a healthy ovum, here is some information about a healthy sperm which is equally important.

Male Reproductive Cell

The male reproductive cell is known as sperm *(shukranu)* and its health is equally important for conception of a fine baby. The main causes of male infertility area are low sperm count, total absence of sperm, and hereditary defects in the production of sperm.

According to Ayurveda, the nature of sperm is 'mild & cooling' and one must take care to protect it against high temperature.

According to Astangasangaraha (an ancient text), healthy semen is mild, well-lubricated, thick in nature, sweet, white in color, honey-like in smell, ample in quantity and resembles ghee, oil or honey.

Signs of imbalance in Semen

Dosha imbalance	Semen imbalance
Vata dosha	Semen is scanty, very liquid in nature and ejaculation is delayed and painful
Pitta dosha	Semen is yellow in color, non-viscous in nature and ejaculation is accompanied by a burning sensation
Kapha dosha	Semen is very sticky and heavy in nature and it discharges in excessive quantity
All three *dosha*	Semen is scanty and bad smelling, accompanied by pus and clots

According to Ayurveda, a conception occurring with imbalanced sperm is rare. But if it does occur, then the chances of a miscarriage are high, or the child might have a short life span, or be weak and unattractive in looks. Thus poor quality of sperm affects not only the father but also his partner and the baby.

Measures to protect semen

Fortunately, there are several measures that a man can do to help protect his semen. Some involve avoiding certain scenarios, while others involve active steps that can be taken.

A man should avoid:

1   Mental stress and staying up till late night badly affect sperm health.
2   Frequent intake of junk food or excessively spicy and oily food, can damage sperm.
3   Excessive heat to the genital area, such as a bath with very hot water, working in very hot environment, frequently having hot steam or sauna baths, wearing tight clothes or placing a laptop directly on lap
4   Addictions like smoking, too much alcohol, even excessive intake of tea can affect the sperm.
5   Inappropriate influences during puberty, such as watching pornographic visuals or magazines, which leads to excessive masturbation, thus causing loss of *shukra dhatu* (sperm) from a very young age. In modern science there is a belief that this is a very natural process and acceptable, but Ayurveda strongly advocates the maximum retention and protection of sperm, which can be achieved by raising *sattva* - which is discussed below.

For healthy semen, it is recommended that a man:

1   Should consider proper nutritional levels in the body, because lack of nutrition results in poor quality of sperm
2   Daily consumption of milk, ghee, milk products, *amla*, *Chyawanprash*, *ashwagandha,* etc are advisable.
3   Raises *sattva* by reading spiritual books, doing yoga or meditation, getting involved in sports, as well as having *sattvik* food and leading a *sattvik* life

The above discussion about the signs, effects and treatment of unhealthy ovum or sperm gives an idea to live a healthy lifestyle. More importantly, it tells what measurements to take to correct any imbalances and have a healthy reproductive system, and be closer to achieving the goal of having a fully healthy baby.

What if you do have a healthy reproductive system?

Now let us look into the second scenario, that you already have a healthy reproductive system. In this case, you might be wondering, why would we need further discussion about it! That's because this topic is about the measures you can take to make your already healthy ovum or sperm healthier! It's like any field of human endeavor. There are good but run-of-the-mill practitioners, and then there are ace practitioners. You want to be in the latter group and thus have the best possible chance of having a baby fully endowed with life's gifts. Here now are some of the things you can do to elevate your reproductive health to the highest levels.

Food

You must consume the food that nourishes the *shukra dhatu* (ovum and sperm). These foods are *sattvik* in nature, and both you and your partner must consume them for at least one month before you plan for a conception.

- **Milk**
  According to Ayurveda, milk is *shukra vardhak*, increases strength and potency and retains youth. To avail the benefits, you and your partner must consume at least one glass of milk every day for a minimum of one month before conception.

- **Ghee** (home-made butter)
  Ghee is also one of the essential food items for nourishing *shukra dhatu*. Both you and your partner should have at least two teaspoons full of ghee every day.

- **Almond**
  Almond has good nutritional value. Soak 4-5 almonds overnight. In the morning peel off their skins and chew them really well so you can absorb all its benefits.

- **Dates, Black Raisins, Leafy Veggies, Spinach, Pomegranate, Soaked Figs**
  These are iron rich foods. Before being pregnant, it is highly recommended that you have very good levels of hemoglobin in your blood. Soaked black raisins also expel excess heat and resolve constipation, which alone are good enough reasons for infertility.

Rejuvenating Herbs

Ayurveda recommends a few herbs which are excellent for *shukra dhatu* and also rejuvenate the whole reproductive system. Some of these are shatavari (Asparagus racemosus), amla, ashwagandha (Withania somnifera), pipli (Indian long pepper), jyeshthamadh (Glycyrrhiza Glabra) and gokshur (Tribulus terrestris).

For Women

Among the herbs above, shatavari is the best herb for women. Consumption of 0.5-1 teaspoon of shatavari powder with a glass of milk works best on a woman's body. It is so safe that anyone can take it without a doctor's prescription. It rejuvenates all the reproductive organs, and is excellent for the formation of breastmilk. Start having it at least three months before you plan for conception, and continue it during full pregnancy for the best result.

[Note: If you have any disease or excessively obese then it is advisable to consult an Ayurvedic Doctor before taking it.]

For Men

Amongst the above herbs *ashwagandha* is the best herb for a male body, and is also very safe. 0.5 teaspoon of *ashwagandha* with sweet milk works great. It rejuvenates the male reproductive system and increases *virya* (*shukra dhatu*). Men should start this herb for a minimum of three months before they plan for a conception.

Yoga

There is no substitute of exercise for a healthy and flexible body. Walking, cycling, swimming or playing any sports are good forms of exercise, but according to Ayurveda, yoga is one of the best forms of exercise. Choose an exercise according to your inclination, but engaging yourself in some form of exercise regularly is highly recommended for the strength and flexibility you'll need when you are pregnant and later a mother.

Here are some yoga postures and *Pranayam* techniques which will make your body strong, healthy and flexible which is necessary before conception. It is recommended to learn yoga from a qualified teacher.

Yoga Postures and *Pranayam*	
Suryanamaskar	*Dhanurasan*
Uttanpadasan	*Butturfly*
Pavnmuktasan	*Paschimotanasan*
Naukasan	*Anulomvilom Pranayam*
Sarvangasan	*Kapalbhati*
Hallasan	*Uddayan Bandha*
Bhujangasan	*Om* Chanting

1.3 Mental Preparation

You must be wondering what mental preparation means! Does it mean that both partners must be mentally ready for having a child? Yes, of course, both mother and father should be mentally prepared for taking the responsibility of a child before planning for it. But that is not enough. Ayurveda considers a deeper meaning in this respect. I personally believe that this is supremely important and this description is only given by Ayurveda!

According to Ayurveda, the *prakruti* (constitution) of the embryo is not decided by God, but by its parents. Yes, what kind of a child you want is in your hands! The *prakruti* is made up of the physical, mental and spiritual states of the embryo. If you want your child to be physically healthy, strong and attractive individual, mentally courageous and firm, as well as spiritually enlightened, pure, calm and a satisfied soul, that also with a good fortune, positive energy and *guna*... then it is in your hands to produce this kind of creation.

According to Ayurveda, your *karma* (deeds) affects your *maan* (mind). *Maan* affects the state of the body, and the state of the body affects the quality of the *shukra dhatu* (ovum and sperm), which obviously directly affects the future child.

Thus, it is logical that the embryo contains all the negative and positive energies possessed by both parents just before the conception. And thus the *prakruti* of the embryo is decided. So, in simple words the physical, mental and spiritual qualities of the embryo depend on the physical, mental and spiritual well-being of both parents.

We've already discussed physical well-being in the earlier topics in this chapter, we'll now talk about the details of mental and spiritual well-being. Again Ayurveda has useful advice in this regard, by indicating a few rules to be followed by both parents for a few months before they plan for conception.

- Try to be punctual with your day to day work and try to be firm in your decisions. Get up early in the morning. Do some exercise, walking and yoga.
- Invest time in prayer and some spiritual reading or *satsang* (spiritual/philosophical discussions).
- Take three meals a day, with regular timing and consume *sattvik* diet. Avoid junk food, very spicy or deep fried food.
- Strictly avoid addictions like smoking, tobacco, alcohol, drugs and excessive consumptions of tea or coffee.
- If your life is stressful, then try to de-stress yourself with the help of music, massage, aroma therapy, or meditation (which works miraculously).
- Don't read or watch any kind of pornographic material that provokes your sexual craving.

- If you have any negative emotions like hatred, anger, jealousy, anxiety, sorrow, or disappointment, then cleanse these emotions from your mind, replacing them with love, forgiveness, satisfaction, peace, happiness and hope.
- If you have any physical illness, then treat it with the help of a good Ayurvedic doctor (*Vaidya*).
- Observe celibacy for one month before the actual *garbhadhan* (conception) to protect and strengthen the *shukra dhatu*.

Thus by achieving firmness, punctuality, courage, peace, happiness, satisfaction, spirituality and all positive energy within both of you, you can transfer these to your child. It is as simple as that.

Indeed, this is such a wonderful science!

For all these processes, just make your own choice of time span you want to practice them, can be 1 month, 6 months or 12 months ... anything. Just give your best to get the best.

1.4   Creating Healthy Surroundings and Atmosphere

The fusion of ovum and sperm with the addition of *pran tatva* creates an individual human being. In Ayurveda, Acharya Charaka from ancient times, also describes the atmosphere in which the conception should occur. So, let's take a small journey into this wondrous topic.

An Ideal Age for Reproduction

According to Indian mythology, during the first quarter of life (i.e. first 25 years of life), man should keep *brahamcharya* (bachelorhood), not only physically but also mentally. This is the time for education and learning, and then after this period, one is eligible for marriage and can enter in to *gruhsthashram*.

According to Ayurveda, the best age for the best production (conception) is 25 years for men and 16 years for women. Even though legally the age for marriage is 21 for men and 18 years for women, you must consider the above criteria when planning for a conception.

Nowadays in India, women usually marry at 23 to 27 years of age, so generally, the ideal time for pregnancy is one or one-and-half year after marriage. That way the couple have time to know and understand each other well. Note though, that this is not a rule, but a general advice.

The maximum age limit for having a child is 65 to 70 years for a man, if he has taken healthy measures to protect his semen from an early age. And it is 35 years for a woman, as it involves many factors like the elasticity and strength of the uterus, general health, period cycle etc. But if you want to conceive after 35 years, you must not lose courage! Instead, take Ayurvedic advice and all the healthy measures that a good Ayurvedic doctor (*Vaidya*) can give you.

Ayurveda also indicates that you and your partner should not be from the same *gotra* (clan), such as marriage between cousins, etc. Because the chromosomes from the same family are very similar and can't match properly, there are higher chances of disorder in the child.

Willingness

Man must keep in mind that a woman is not always in a ready and charged mode for sexual activity as he generally is. According to Ayurveda, women have highs-and-lows in their moods for sexual activity, while men are generally in a high mood. So, when they intend to go for a conception they must come together when each is equally willing for sexual intercourse. It must not be without consent or a forced activity.

Specifically, Ayurveda also indicates the duration when women generally have high moods for sexual activity. It is 2-3 days prior to her period cycle, and also from the first day of the period up to the sixteenth night. These are also considered to be the most fertile days for conception, but they should not go for sexual intercourse when her period is on. Woman's mood may differ, but still, they must come together when they are equally willing, for life-long benefit of the fetus, as well as for themselves on this momentous occasion.

The Bedroom

The bedroom in which the conception is to take place should be clean, calm, cozy and full of positive vibrations. You can even create *dhoop* (a smoke with fragrant and purifying herbs) in it. The bed should be covered with a clean and light, or calm-colored bed spread. You can even light a *diya* (lamp) in the bedroom for a calm and enlightened atmosphere. An aroma lamp is also a wonderful idea to make your mind relaxed and light.

Both of you should wear white or nice bright color clothes. Very dark colored clothes shouldn't be worn as they provoke the mind.

Thus you can do whatever you like, using your own creativity, to create a nice, calm, pure and positive atmosphere in your bedroom, so that it will be a suitable place for your planned conception, a place of pure positive vibrations and love.

One more thing Ayurveda adds is that the place where conception occurs should be familiar. It should not occur in any new, foreign place, such as on your honeymoon, where it may lack good hygiene and authentic positive vibrations.

1.5   Garbhadhan

So far we discussed what can be done to strengthen physical, mental and spiritual health, so that, with the assistance of these guidelines, you are now prepared for *garbhadhan* (conception).

So ... fill your mind and body with positive and pure energies, make your soul lighten, and let's talk about the *garbhadhan vidhi* (conception process).

When a woman becomes *rutumati* and after her *rutusnan*, she gets ready for sexual intercourse with the intention of a conception, and the man should give his sperm to her through intercourse. When she accepts the sperm in her body, it is called *garbhadhan*.

You must be wondering. Here is the terminology to help you to understand what was just described.

Terminology

Rutumati	A woman who is having her period
Rutusnan	The bath taken after three days of a woman's period
Rutukaal	The most fertile period in the woman's monthly cycle. *Rutukaal* extends from the 1st day of menstruation onwards to the 16th night after menstruation began.
	It means that a total of these 16 nights are the most fertile nights. And during this period, if sexual intercourse takes place, the chances of conception are higher (one must avoid sexual activity till menstrual cycle is on).

Acharya Sushrut has explained the Garbhadhan vidhi (process) in following words.

ततोऽपहान्हे पुमान मासं ब्रह्मचारी सर्पीः क्षीराभ्यां
शाल्योदन भुक्त्वा मासं ब्रह्मचारिनि तैलस्निग्धां
तलमासोत्तराहारां नारीमुपेयाद्रातौ सामादिभिर्विश्वास्य विकल्पयेवं
चतुर्थ्यांष्टष्ठवाष्ष्ट्यां दशम्यां द्वादश्यां चोपेयादिति पुत्रकामः ॥

Meaning: After observing one month of celibacy man should take body massage with ghee, and consume ghee, rice and milk as part of his meal. And after observing one month of celibacy, woman should take a body massage with oil, and consume food prepared from *urad dal (black or white lentil)* (such as *urad ladoo* or any preparation using it) for a meal.

Thus, each of them gets ready for conception.

In the night with full willingness and with love the man who desires to have a child should bring the woman to an equal level of willingness and then they should go for sexual intercourse.

Ayurveda says one must have a *sattvik* diet on the *garbhadhan* day. *Rajsik* and *tamsik* diets badly affect your mind and body. The *tamshik* diet, for example, changes sexual desire into sexual craving, by simply provoking the mind. Ghee, milk and rice are of a *sattvik* nature, and also rejuvenate the sperm, while oil and *urad dal* strengthen the ovum. That's why the *sattvik* diet is desirable.

The ideal time for conception

Rutukaal is the most fertile period for conception. But remember that intercourse must not take place till the blood flow persists. If both partners come together before that there is no possibility for conception, instead could be detrimental to health of both.

So to conceive a strong and healthy child of the best quality, the ideal time for *garbhadhan* is few days after menstruation, specifically from the 8th day to the 16th night. Moreover, it is better to choose a night as late as possible before the 16th night, because after the 16th night it is rare for a conception to take place. Even if it occurs there is a possibility that the resulting child could be weak, less good looking, with a low immune system and so on. The reason behind this, is that after the 16th night the cervix starts to contract and thus become a hindrance to conception.

According to Ayurveda, sexual intercourse should take place only at night, during the 2nd *prahar*, which is before 1.30 to 2 am. Ayurveda does not advise conception occurring during daytime.

Before the sexual intercourse you and your partner should not be thirsty, hungry, stressed, exhausted, overly eaten or up till late night. Ideally, both the couple should be free from all kinds of stress, anxiety, worry, anger, sadness, negative thoughts etc.

The constitution of the child also depends on the weather and season during which *garbhadhan* occurs. In winter (*hemant* and *shishir*) physical strength is at its peak, so generally this is the ideal time for conception.

How to Calculate the 1st Day

Calculating the 1st day can be a bit tricky sometimes. If menstrual bleeding starts at night rather than during daytime, Ayurveda provides following description to determine the first day:

- Divide the night into three part from sunset to sunrise.
- If you start bleeding in the first two parts, then call that the 1st day.
- If you start bleeding in the third part, then call the next day the 1st day.

For example

1. If sunset on Monday is at 7 pm and sunrise on Tuesday is 7 am, the night is 12 hours long.
   o Divide the 12 hours into three parts, which means the first 2 parts equal 8 hours.
   o If you start bleeding before 3 am on Tuesday, consider Monday as your 1st day.
   o If you start bleeding after 3 am on Tuesday, consider Tuesday as your 1st day.

2. Sometimes, even this can be tricky, if for example, the duration of sunset to sunrise is 11 hours. Each part then becomes 3 hours 40 minutes. So if you need to make this kind of calculation, you need to be very accurate, even considering something as small as a minute.

1.6   What Do You Want? A Baby Boy? Or A Baby Girl?

Ayurveda is such an intriguing science, it says that it is in your hands to decide the gender of the embryo! Acharya Sushrut explains this in following words:

युग्मेषु तु पुमान् प्रोक्तो दिवसेष्वयथाङ्बला ।
पुष्णकाले शुचोस्तस्मादपास्यार्थी स्त्रीयं व्रजेत् ॥

Meaning: After *rutusnan*, if sexual intercourse takes place during an even number night, such as 6th, 8th, 10th, 12th, or 16th night, the couple will create a baby boy. And if the couple desires a baby girl, they should go for any odd numbered night, like the 5th, 7th, 9th or 15th.

Naturally the question arises, why is this so? Is it something important to do with the night? Or are there physical reasons for it? The answer is to do with the following *Sanskrit shloka*.

आधिक्ये रजस: कन्या पुत्र: शुक्राधिके भवेत् ।

The above *Sanskrit shloka* refers to the facts that:
* When the ovum is stronger, it produces a baby girl.
* When the sperm is stronger, it produces a baby boy.

So it means that a physical factor is more important. In the even numbered nights (6th, 8th, etc.) the woman's ovum gets a little weaker, so the man's sperm is relatively stronger, and that's why they produce a baby boy. Reverse is the case for odd numbered nights, giving more probability for a baby girl.

It's not that simple though, just selecting a day is not enough. Ancient Yoga also provides some insights into this. Yoga says that the *swar* which is running during conception also determines the sex of the child.

The word *swar* refers to *surya nadi* (which is the right nostril running) and *chandra nadi* (the left nostril running). You can easily check which of your nostrils is running by putting your finger near to each nostril and exhaling. Where you feel a good force of exhalation, is the nostril that is running.

Now if a man with his *surya nadi* running goes for sexual intercourse and if a conception occurs, the resulting child will be baby boy; and with *chandra nadi* the resulting child will be a baby girl.

There are many ways to activate the *nadi* of your choice. The easiest way is to lie down on the lateral side opposite the *nadi* you want to activate for 10-15 minutes.

For example

- If one wants to activate his *surya nadi* (right nostril), then he should lie down on his left lateral side for 10-15 minutes so his right nostril will start working, and vice versa.
- It is recommended for the man to check his nostril before sexual intercourse.

So, in essence, you need to consider two things: the selection of the day, and the selection of the *nadi swar*.

- To have a baby boy:
  - Conception should occur in any of the even numbered nights, such as the 6th, 8th, 10th, 12th, 14th or 16th night.
  - Man should go for sexual intercourse after activating his *surya nadi*.

- To have a baby girl:
  - Conception should occur in any of the odd numbered nights, such as the 7th, 9th, 11th, 13th or 15th night.
  - Man should go for sexual intercourse after activating his *chandra nadi*.

(Please note that *swar* selection is required only by the man, not by the woman.)

Please do not take this information wrongly! We are educated people and are living in a beautiful society where both baby boys and baby girls are equally accepted and loved.

....

Here, we conclude the chapter on preparing for pregnancy. If you are planning a conception sometime in the future, hopefully you have found out things that you can start now. Perhaps there are some behaviors or habits that you can now see it would be better to drop – and substitute with something more nourishing to your health and thereby to the health of the child you will eventually have. Perhaps it is just a matter of fine-tuning the way you currently live to capitalize on the good that's already there.

We turn next to the vital care of the mother during her pregnancy, care that has to provide for the health of both her precious baby in-utero and herself.

Care during Pregnancy

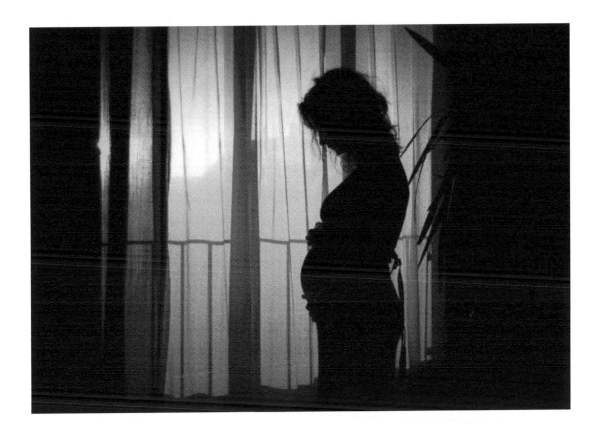

Congratulations!!! You have conceived. I am sure when you found out that you are pregnant; your heart must have missed a beat. The start of a pregnancy is one of the most unforgettable moments consisting of excitement, happiness, a little hesitation, anxiety and tension with lots of doubts in mind.

Calm down yourself. Take a deep breath. In this section we'll talk about all the minor details about pregnancy like the physical changes in your body during pregnancy, common problems during pregnancy and their treatment, food, exercise and many more things. I believe you must spend your pregnancy with adequate knowledge and full of joy because this is one of the most beautiful time of life, after which you will get the best gift in the world.

So ... roll up your sleeves and make up your mind to enjoy this time in full health, peace and calmness that anyone has ever possessed.

2.1 Early Signs of Pregnancy

Generally, an intuitive woman may immediately sense that she has conceived. But most women only begin to suspect that they may be pregnant after missing a period. Still, by then they have already passed 14-15 days.

Acharya Charaka has indicated signs of early pregnancy by following words:

निष्ठो विका गौरव भऽग्साद:
तन्द्रा प्रहर्षो ह्रदयव्यथा च |
तृषिश्च बीजग्रहणं च योग्या
गर्भस्या सघाऽनुगतस्य लिंगम् |

Here are the signs of early pregnancy.

- Heaviness in the body, especially on thighs
- Nausea, vomiting, dizziness, low energy
- Fatigue and weakness
- Lots of saliva in mouth, palpitations, heartburn
- Dislike of food and sexual activity
- Aversion to strong smells.
- Feeling of deep inner satisfaction
- Morning sickness

Not all women have all these symptoms. Some women have only a few of them, and a few blessed ones have none at all! It's always best to get as clean and healthy as possible both mentally and physically before conception so your pregnancy goes more smoothly. However, it also depends on the constitution both you and your fetus have.

According to Acharya Charka, the Father of Medicine in Ayurveda, a pregnant woman is like a pot filled with oil till the brim which requires an absolutely steady hand to take it from one place to another. She must aim to take great care of both her fetus and herself. In his text, *Charak Samhita,* there are some dos and don'ts for pregnant women which are profoundly desirable to carry out all the way through the pregnancy. That way she maximizes the chances for an absolutely healthy pregnancy along with the health benefits for her fetus and herself.

Dos ...

1. Sleep on both sides as far as possible, using both equally, and not favoring either one excessively. If you sleep on your back, there are chances that the umbilical cord will twine itself around the neck of the fetus.
2. Wear loose and comfortable garments, thus avoiding tight fitting clothes like jeans and skirts as they will restrict a proper blood flow. Wear flat-heeled sandals, thus avoiding high-heeled ones. Wear a comfortable fitted bra, not a tight one.
3. You may feel lazy and heavy during your pregnancy, but keep yourself active by doing all your day-to-day tasks. It generates good blood circulation in the body and a good level of flexibility in your muscles.
4. Remain happy and joyful. Involve yourself in reading good books, attaining *satsang*, doing meditation and yoga to keep yourself calm, at peace and enlightened. Do not watch or read things which create fear, anxiety, negativity or grief in you, as they directly affect the mind of the fetus.

And Don'ts ...

1. Do not suppress any natural urges like urination, defecation or flatulence, as it could result in an imbalance of *vata dosha*. Suppression of an urge to urinate may cause a urinary tract infection or pain in your abdomen. Suppression of defecation may cause loss of appetite, constipation and gas formation. Suppression of flatulence may cause nausea, belching or heartburn.
2. Avoid travelling or having to ride on vehicles that vibrate a lot. Avoid jerks and bumps. Don't travel long distances during the first trimester and the last two months. Travel during the remaining four months only if it is necessary – and ensure you have a very comfortable journey.
3. Avoid excessive physical work, inappropriate exercise, gym exercises, vigorous aerobics, strenuous swimming or cycling.
4. Do not eat food that is too spicy, too hot or too pungent. Avoid unhealthy food. Excessive or very little consumption of food is not advisable, just eat according to your appetite. Be rest assured that you don't need to eat for two – that is just a myth. Avoid refined flour, uncooked salt, excessive white sugar.
5. Give up smoking, alcohol, and excessive tea or coffee entirely.
6. Avoid loud or disturbing noises. Don't look into the depths of a well, or valley, or down from the top of the high-rise building as these could cause fear or a physical jolt which could harm the fetus.
7. Don't stay up late at night or sleep during the day, since late night imbalances *vata* in your mind and body, and sleeping during day imbalances *kapha* in the body. Resting in the afternoon is acceptable, but deep sleep is not.
8. Avoid sexual intercourse throughout your pregnancy, this being strictly prohibited by Ayurveda in the first and last trimesters.

2.2   Monthly development of fetus and special diet for each month

5000 years ago when there were no laboratory instruments for investigation, Ayurveda described the development of the fetus for each month in its mother's womb, and it's so accurate. What breathtaking science the Ayurveda is!

So here we'll outline the monthly development of the fetus according to both Ayurveda and modern science. And we will also discuss the special diet you as a mother-to-be should consume month by month to add to the health of both your fetus and yourself.

1ˢᵗ Month

According to Ayurveda

स सर्वगुणवान् गर्भत्वम् आपन्न:
प्रधमं मासि संमुच्छित: सर्वधातुकलुषीकृत:
खेतभुतो भवत्यव्यक्तविग्रह: सत् असत् भूताऽगवयव: ॥

(From Charaka Sharirshthan)

Translation:
When the soul (*atma*) comes in a womb, it emerges in five elements (*panchmahabhoot*) that creates a life. In the first month the embryo resembles a ball of mucus.

तत्र प्रथमे मासि कल्लं जायते ।

(From Sushrut Sharirthan)

Translation:
In the first month the embryo resembles a morula (an early stage of embryo).

According to modern science

The embryo is about 0.6 cm (0.25 inches) long. Within 18-25 days after fertilization its developing heart begins to beat. Then four small buds become visible, which are its embryonic arms and legs.

Special Diet in the First Month

It is good to consume a sweet and cooling liquid diet. So it is good to sip on milk at room temperature throughout the day, after having been boiled earlier.

2nd Month

According to Ayurveda

दितेये मासी घन: संपधेते
पिण्ड: पेशी अर्बुदम वा
तत्र घन: पुरुष, पेशी स्त्री, अर्बुद नपुंसक्म ॥

(From Charak Sharirshthan)

Translation:
In the second month the embryo increases in density and slowly becomes round, oval or tear-drop shaped. If it's a round shape, it means it's a baby boy; if oval shaped, it's a baby girl.

According to modern science

The embryo is about 3 cm (1.2 inches) long and weighs about 1 gm (0.03 ounces). The eyes have started to develop, but the distance between two eyes is more than required. Its nose has been formed, but it is still flat. Its arms and legs are well developed now and its fingers are also formed. In this month the process of forming internal organs has also started.

Special diet in the second month

It is good to consume any one of these cooling and sweet-tasting herbs, such as shatavari, bala, gokshur and vidari with boiled milk that has cooled down.

3rd Month

According to Ayurveda

तृतीये मासी सर्वेन्दियाणि
सर्वाॱग अवयनश्च
यौगपधेन अभिनिर्वतंन्ते ।

(From Charaka Sharirshthan)

Translation:
In the third month all the senses and organs start forming.

तृतीये हस्तपादशिरशांग सन्य
पिंडिक्का निर्वतन्ते ᳵगपत्यंᳵग
विभागश्च सूक्ष्मो भवति ।

(From Sushrut Sharirthan)

Translation:
The tiny round fetus appears to have five different parts, a tail, two arms and two legs. It has organs and its senses are developing at a micro level.

According to modern science
The fetus is about 7.5 cm (3 inches) long and weighs about 30 gm (1 ounce). The eyes are completely formed. The nose is also taking shape. The nails have started forming. Its heartbeat can be detected. Urine starts to form, which means its urinary system has started functioning. And the fetus begins to move, but that can't be felt yet by the mother.

Special diet in the third month
It is good to have milk with rice (kheer), as well as warm milk with 2 tsp of ghee and 1 tsp of honey.

4th Month

According to Ayurveda

चतुर्थे मासि स्थिरत्वम् आपध्यते गर्भः ||

(From Charaka Sharirshthan)

Translation:
In the fourth month the fetus becomes stable, which means there is less chance for miscarriage as its placenta has developed fully.

चतुर्थे सर्वाऽगप्रत्यऽग
विभाग प्रत्यक्तो भवति
गर्भे हृदय प्रत्यक्ति भवति |

(From Sushrut Sharirthan)

Translation:
In the fourth month all the parts of the body are defined better, and particularly the heart can be experienced, which means the mother has two hearts and the fetus expresses its wishes through the mother. According to Ayurveda, one must fulfill these wishes if they are genuine.

According to modern science
The fetus is about 18 cm (7 inches) long and weighs about 100 gm (3.5 ounces). In this month the head is large in proportion to the rest of the body. Its facial features now appear human. Hairs start to grow on its head. The skin color is bright pink.

Special diet in the fourth month
It is good to consume rice with curd, and every morning it is good to have 1-2 tsp of ghee with crystal sugar (mishri).

5th Month

According to Ayurveda

पंच्यमे मासि गर्भस्य मांस शोणित
उपजयो भवति अधिकम् अन्येभ्यो मासेभ्यो: ॥

(From Charaka Sharirshthan)

Translation:
In this month the maximum development of mansa dhatu (muscles) and rakta dhatu (blood) occurs compared to the other months.

पंच्यमे मन: प्रतिबुध्धतरं भवति ।

(From Sushrut Sharirthan)

Translation:
In the fifth month the mind of the fetus is fully developed, which means that now the child is very sensitive to its surroundings and the various feelings its mother has.

According to modern science
The fetus is 25-30 cm (9.8-11.8 inches) long and weighs 200-450 gm (7-15.8 ounces). Its head is less disproportionate to the rest of its body now. Its body hair started growing. Kicking or movement will be felt by the mother.

Special diet in the fifth month
It is good to consume milk and rice preparation, like kheer and also 7-8 tsp of ghee throughout the whole day. (You also need to be active enough to digest this food.)

6th Month

According to Ayurveda

षष्ठे मासि गर्भस्य बलवर्णोपचयो भवति
अधिकं अन्येभ्यो मासेभ्य: |

(From Charak Sharirshthan)

Translation:
In the sixth month development of strength and complexion occurs, which means you will feel more baby's movement and the skin of the child will radiate. You may also feel weak during this month.

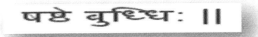

(From Sushrut Sharirsthan)

Translation:
In the sixth month the intelligence (*buddhi*) develops.

According to modern science
The fetus is 27-35 cm (10.6-13.7 inches) long and weighs 550-800 gm (1.25-1.75 pounds). The head continues to become even less disproportionate in size to the rest of the body. Its eyelids separate and the eye lenses appear. Its skin becomes pink.

Special diet in the sixth month
It is good to consume ghee and rice in this month. Ghee with the herb, shatavari is good in the morning on an empty stomach. This is the time where the complexion of the child develops so it's good to consume saffron with milk, buttermilk, young coconut water, kheer, etc.

7th Month

According to Ayurveda

सप्तमे मासे गर्भ: सर्वेभावै: आप्याप्यते ॥

(From Charaka Sharirsthan)

Translation:
In the seventh month all the systems and dhatus are fully developed.

सप्तमे सर्वाऽङ्गप्रत्यङ्ग विभाग: प्रव्यक्तर: ।

(From Sushrut Sharirsthan)

Translation:
In the seventh month all the organs are essentially developed.

According to modern science
The fetus is 32-42 cm (12.6-16.5 inches) long and weighs 1.1-1.35 kg (2.5-3 pounds). The head and body are now more proportionate.

Special diet in the seventh month
Continue the diet from the sixth month.

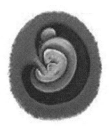

1 month

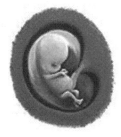

2 month

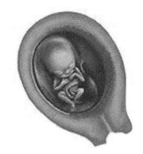

3 month

8th Month

According to Ayurveda

अष्टमे मासे गर्भश्च मातृतो
गर्भच्च माता रसहारिणिभी:
संवाहिनीभि: मुहु: मुहुर: ओज:
परस्परत आददाते गर्भस्या संपूर्णत्यात्...||

(From Charaka Sharirsthan)

Translation:
Wise Vaidya (Ayurvedic doctors) believes that this month is not suitable for delivery, as the *ojas* (life energy) is not stable in this month. It alternates between the mother and the fetus. So, if premature labor occurs, the life of the one lacking ojas at the time may be in jeopardy.
(As the *ojas* flows alternatively to the mother and then to the fetus, you may feel extremely happy and enthusiastic when it flows into you, and tired and drained when it does not.)

According to modern science
The fetus is 41-45 cm (16-17.75 inches) long and weighs 2-2.3 kg (4.5-5 pounds). Fat is deposited and chances of survival are much greater at the end of the 8th month.

Special diet in the eighth month
In this month consume rice with milk and sugar (kheer).

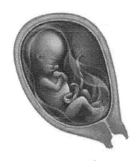
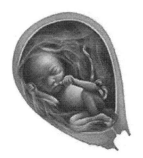
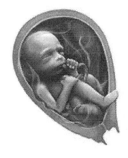

4 month   5 month   6 month

9th Month

According to Ayurveda

तस्मित्रेकदिवसतिक्रान्तेडपि नवमं मासं उपादाय प्रसवकालं
इत्याहुरादशमान् मासात् ।

(From Charaka Sharirshthan)

Translation:

As the eighth month ends and the ninth month starts, it is the right time for your delivery. By now the fetus has developed completely.

(A delay in delivery is not desirable as the placenta which nourishes the fetus starts degenerating. So if you know the exact day of conception, you can easily calculate the day of delivery. Labor starts generally around the 280th day)

According to modern science

The fetus is about 50 cm (19.5 inches) long and weighs 3.2-3.4 kg (6.25-6.75 pounds.

Special diet in the ninth month

Consume milk + rice + ghee.

Castor oil also works well in this month, 5-6 days prior to your due date for labor.

Castor oil preparation

Take half a cup of milk + 2 pinches of dry ginger powder + gud (jaggery) according to taste. Boil this mixture. Take it off the flame, and then add 1-2 tsp of castor oil and have the mixture hot.

This preparation resolves constipation and balances apan vayu (situated in the lower part of the belly) which is required for normal delivery and smooth labor. It also has labor inducing property.

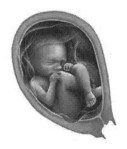 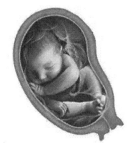 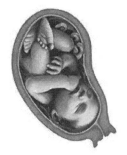

7 month   8 month   9 month

2.3 Essential Nutrition

The food that you consume throughout pregnancy impacts a lot on the nature of pregnancy , the health of the fetus and the development of breast milk. According to Ayurveda, the mother-to-be should eat only such food that:

1. Keeps her pregnancy healthy and nourishes her body.
2. Nourishes and develops the fetus.
3. Generates a good quantity and quality of breast milk.

So let's have a look at some essential nutrition and food that is best to consume during pregnancy.

Iron

One of the inevitable factors for forming blood is iron. All born babies are fed exclusively on breast milk for almost a year, but breastmilk has very low levels of iron. However, nature has a fascinating arrangement! The fetus absorbs a good amount of iron from its mother's body while it is in her uterus which it stores in its liver for later use. So, the mother-to-be must consume a good amount of iron during pregnancy.

Good sources of iron are *neem* leaves, mint (*pudina)*, coriander, soybean, sesame (*til)*, raisins, dates, leafy vegetables especially spinach, apricot, pomegranate, beetroot, jaggery water, etc.

Jaggery water preparation

Soak a small amount of jaggery (a concentrated product of cane sugar or palm sap) in water for a few hours. Let it dilute and drink this water.

A deficiency of iron can cause weakness, fatigue, loss of luster, low weight of the fetus, complications during labor, and heart palpitations and it leaves you without enthusiasm for life.

Vitamin C

Vitamin C is essential for the optimum absorption of iron. Lemon, Indian gooseberry (*amla)*, orange, tomato, spinach (*palak)*, basil (*tulsi)*, and cauliflower are good sources of Vitamin C.

Vitamin E

There is enough evidence to say that a woman with a tendency of miscarriage, can have a normal delivery by having a good amount of Vitamin E. It helps to prevent premature rupture of the amniotic sack and also increases the quality of amniotic fluid.

Good sources of Vitamin E are spinach (*palak*), beans, sprouts (especially mung), jaggery water, rice, parsley, broccoli, etc.

Calcium

During pregnancy the mother's body demands more calcium, because the developing fetus absorbs calcium from its mother's body to form strong bones and teeth, and to grow a healthy heart, nerves, muscles and the blood's clotting ability. So if you don't have enough calcium, the fetus draws it from your bones, which may impair your own health later on.

Milk is the best source for calcium. It helps to develop the *dhatus* (Ayurveda's seven fundamental parts of the body) and strong bones of the fetus. According to Ayurveda, it increases the *ojas*. 2-3 glasses of milk per day works very well during pregnancy. It is important that the milk be pure and fresh. Pasteurized milk is also safe, but not any others like ultra-heated milk or vitamin enriched milk.

Other dairy products like yogurt, cottage cheese, buttermilk, ghee, wheat, finger millet (*raagi*), and pulses like *mung dhal* or *toor dhal* and so on are good sources of calcium.

A deficiency of calcium may cause weakness, back-pain, muscle cramps and joint pain.

Glucose

In the first six months of the pregnancy, the fetus requires a lot of glucose. At that time if the mother's liver lacks glycogen then her liver becomes weak, and one of the main function of liver is to purify blood, this could result into contamination of blood.

Good sources of glucose are jaggery water, honey, sugarcane juice and dates. And these have the added benefit of solving the problem of vomiting.

But during the last trimester all these items should be restricted to a minimum quantity and should be replaced with milk and fruits.

Protein

Protein is not only required for the growth of the fetus but also to treat all the wear and tear in your body, especially during the second and third trimesters when the fetus is growing at a faster rate.

All pulses are great sources of protein, so are sprouts, almond, peanuts, black chickpeas (*deshi chana*), as well as combinations of pulses + rice or pulses + wheat.

Summary

This is a lot of information on the nutrition required. And of course, you'll be wanting to follow it throughout your pregnancy, as it's crucial for both your darling growing fetus and the mother-to-be – you, yourself. So here is the summary that can be more easily referred to and used.

Say a big YES to:

It is vital that you eat according to your hunger. It is myth that you need to eat for two, but on the other hand, eating food without hunger leads to constipation, indigestion, vomiting, heaviness, swelling and gas formation.

It is advisable to finish your dinner by 7 at night, but after that you can have fruit or milk if you feel hungry.

- Say a big, big yes to milk, ghee, buttermilk, and *paneer* (cottage cheese).
- Add at least two fruits from grapes, apple, pomegranate, Indian gooseberries (*amla*), orange, and sweet lime to your diet each day. Also it is recommended that these fruits be consumed in their season when they are easily available in natural form.
- Consume pineapple, strawberry and cherry only occasionally.
- Include fresh fruit juice in your diet, such as lemon juice, orange juice or sweet lime juice.
- Include fresh coconut water in your diet too, it is another healthy drink that ensures your uterus has adequate amniotic fluid, however drink it before 3pm as it may form gas if it is consumed during evening. You can also have young coconut pulp (*malai*) and ripe coconut to make the skin of both your fetus and yourself glowing and healthy.
- You can have mango pulp but with 2-3 tsp of ghee and a pinch of *suthi* (dried ginger powder) so it does not aggravate your *pitta dosha*. One bowl per day is enough.
- Almond, raisins and dry dates work excellent during pregnancy. Soak 4-5 almonds, 10-12 black raisins and 1-2 dry dates for 5-6 hours and then consume them. Soaked and peeled almond nourishes the brain of the developing fetus. Soaked black raisins expels excess heat, corrects bowel movement and also improves the hemoglobin level. Soaked dry dates help the fetus to gain weight.
- Consume the nutritious herbs *brahmi* ("Bacopa monnieri") and *shatavari* ("Asparagus racemosus"). 1 tsp of each can be taken either together or separately with about 1 cup of milk. *Brahmi* strengthens the nervous system and nourishes the brain of the fetus, whereas *shatavari* helps to improve the quantity and quality of mother's breast milk as well as rejuvenates her reproductive system.

Say a Big NO to:

- Refined flour (*maida*) in the form of breads, pizza, biscuits, cakes and bakery products is a big, big NO.
- Papaya may induce miscarriage, so it must never be consumed during pregnancy.
- Raw green mangoes and tamarind should be avoided as they increase *pitta* (heat) in the body. If you crave them, consume as little as possible, just enough to satisfy your taste buds.
- Street food and stale food should not be eaten.
- Tea, coffee, cold drinks, chocolate, aerated drinks, smoking, and alcohol are to be avoided, as caffeine and tannin causes insomnia, acidity and anxiety.
- White sugar should to be avoided whenever possible and should be replaced with honey, jaggary or crystalized sugar (*mishry*)
- Very spicy, hot and deep fried food must be avoided.

2.4 Some Essential Activities

Lot of changes take place in your body when you are a mother-to-be! You would want your pregnancy and labor to go smoothly, as well as good health of yourself and the baby after delivery. Here are some essential activities advised by Ayurveda that should be a part of your routine in order to respond effectively to those changes.

Stretch Marks

During pregnancy the breast, navel, lower abdominal, thighs and thigh joints undergo numerous changes, and because of these they can become itchy too. But you should not scratch, because your nails will damage the skin and scratching it will develop stretch marks. If itching becomes unbearable, then you can use cotton or muslin cloth, dipped in hot water mixed with cooking soda or borax powder and lightly massage the area to bring relief.

For abdominal stretch marks regular massage with oil works well. You can even do oil massage lightly twice or thrice a day, if your skin is very dry.

Massage

You can practice daily self-massage with warm sesame oil or any herbal oil such as Dhanwantharam Thailam, in a warm, quiet room with pleasant music playing. Use your open palm rather than your fingertips, and apply long strokes along your long bones and circular strokes around your joints. Spend more time on any painful areas, but be careful to be gentle on your abdominal region where it is best to softly stroke in a clockwise direction around your naval.

This reduces stress marks, soothes the neuromuscular system, and aids assimilation and elimination whilst reducing leg swelling and varicosities.

Care of the breasts

Your breasts and nipples undergo lots of changes during pregnancy too. They start to increase in size, so you should wear a very comfortable fitted bra and avoid a bra that is even slightly tight, as it restricts the circulation of blood and also the production of milk. From the first day you should start massaging your breasts lightly with *til* (sesame) oil till the ninth month. In the last trimester along with massage you should also apply castor oil to your nipples. Massage helps to reduce sagging of the breasts and keeps them soft and supple and prevents cracks and cuts.

Yoga and Meditation

Yoga helps miraculously during pregnancy by contributing to a healthy and smooth pregnancy and an easy labor. You must make a point of practicing yoga regularly throughout your pregnancy to avail all the benefits. You can find a detailed description of the best yoga *asanas* to be done during pregnancy in the next chapter.

Meditation also works excellently during pregnancy, by keeping your mind calm, controlled and relaxed. It also helps reduce stress outstandingly for working women. There are lots of types of meditation, but simply it means concentrating your mind on a single thing, on your breath, for instance, or on 'Om' chanting being played on CD/DVD or youtube. To pamper yourself even more thoroughly, you may use an aroma while meditating.

You can even practice the extraordinarily deep relaxation technique of Yoga Nidra, which is sometimes called 'psychic sleep'.

Behavior

Acharya Sushrut calls the behavior of the mother-to-be throughout the whole pregnancy as *Garbhini Charya* (pregnant lady behavior). In his program of antenatal care, he recommends that a pregnant woman should:

- Rise early, bath with warm water and wear light colored clothes.
- Perform *puja* or chants/prayer according to her belief.
- Read spiritual books, or books that speak of ethics and morals so as to inculcate good values into the fetus; even the biographies of great personalities are recommended.
- Do not carry heavy loads, and do not talk in a loud voice.
- Do not indulge in anger, fright or other agitating emotions.

- Avoid watching movies and TV serials which are frightening or vulgar, or which make you feel sad, as these will affect the growing fetus.

2.5 Remedies for Common Problems

As a pregnant woman one may face some minor illnesses during the pregnancy. Ayurveda describes some very natural remedies to overcome them.

According to *Charaka Samhita*, the oldest known Ayurvedic text, the medicines prescribed for minor illnesses should be of a mild nature, devoid of side effects and not cause heat in the body.

According to Naturopathy, if you properly cleanse your intestines by having regular and proper bowel movements even old toxicities will be expelled, and if you increase your digestive fire with a *sattvik* diet and lifestyle before a conception, you will not be susceptible to illnesses, or at the least, will face only minimal problems.

You should not have any kind of painkillers or antibiotics as both you and the unborn child will be very susceptible to their side effects. If you really require these medicines, you must consult a doctor.

Here now are some excellent and innocent remedies for common illnesses during pregnancy that you can use when need be.

Constipation

You should not neglect constipation if it occurs frequently. It has lots of nasty and harmful side-effects, such as abdominal pain, backache, leg pain, perhaps even dysentery. Chronic constipation can cause a delayed and painful labor, as a clean and strong intestine is necessary for an easy labor.

Eat only when you are really hungry!

- Banana, butter, ghee, fruits and milk should be added to your regular diet in order to improve your bowel movements.
- In earlier times, there was a ritual of giving 2-3 teaspoons of ghee + a glass of milk at night to pregnant women after the fifth month to make her intestines soft and ready to excrete her feces smoothly.
- *Gulkand* (rose petal jam) + milk works very well during bedtime.

- Raisins + rose petals + crystalized sugar lumps (*mishri* or rock sugar) in an equal quantity with milk once a day. Any time during the day works well, but especially during bedtime.
- *Swadisht Virechan Churna* (an ayurvedic laxative) or *Triphla* can be consumed occasionally.
- 1-1.5 tsp of castor oil with milk, boiled with *suthi* (dried ginger powder) and sugar works really well.
- According to Naturopathy, an enema also works well for treating constipation

Gas, flatulence, abdominal pain or heaviness in the body

These occur because the body has poor digestive fire, and also because of constipation. It is vital to first solve the constipation problem which will in turn help to streamline the digestion process.

- Mixing *Lavanbhaskar Churna* (a compound classical herbal mixture/spice) with buttermilk and consuming it after a meal works well to remove gas or flatulence.
- Fennel seed (*souph*), mint, cardamom (*elaichi)* and ginger are ingredients which increase digestive fire.

Nausea and Vomiting

Nausea or vomiting may start from 2nd month and resolve itself by the end of 4th or 5th month. It occurs from the second month because the embryo increases in density which brings changes in the medulla oblongata (the brain stem which controls the autonomic functions such as breathing and digestion and so on), which affects your breathing and because of this your muscles are stimulated causing nausea or vomiting.

- Squeeze 4 lemons in 150 ml of water, and sip throughout the day to complete it.
- Consume 5 gm of coriander juice diluted with water.
- Have a Hip Bath. It works excellently.
- Consume pomegranate, orange and fig.
- Constipation also causes vomiting so treat it first.
- Soak some *kadiyatu* (Andrographis Paniculata) in water at night, strain it in the morning and add some *mishri* (crystalized sugar lumps/rock sugar) in the water, and have this preparation 2-3 times a day.

Coughing

Coughing occurs when the uterine muscle gets stimulated for no particular reason, which leads to other muscle stimulation and causes coughing. It is better to treat it early on.

- Oily and spicy foods should be completely avoided.
- 0.5-1 tsp of *Sitopaladi churna* (an Ayurvedic medicine) with 1 tsp of honey or 1 cup of milk is very beneficial.
- *Adusol* syrup (an Ayurvedic cough syrup) or *Adusi* leaves (Adhatoda vasica) boiled in water works well.

Acidity or Heartburns

The hormone progesterone, a muscle relaxant, is made in abundance in your body when you are pregnant. It relaxes all the muscles in your body including the valve at the top of your stomach that normally keeps any food you have swallowed and your stomach acid down in your stomach, so when the valve relaxes, stomach acid and sometimes partially digested food can squeeze back up into your esophagus (food pipe). This causes a burning sensation in your chest.

Secondly, as your fetus grows, it needs more space to survive, so the uterus forces your stomach upwards and puts pressure on your digestive tract, causing heartburn.

- Drink coconut water regularly to soothe heartburn and act as a natural neutralizer for any acid, but do so before 3 pm.
- Doing *Shitali pranayam* is very helpful – please check Chapter 3 for this.
- Drink 8-10 glasses of water every day.
- Avoid spicy, oily and acidic foods.
- Consume *gulkand* (rose petal jam), soaked raisins, mishri, etc.

Swelling (edema)

Swollen feet are a common occurrence towards the ends of the third trimester. Swelling (edema) occurs because your body is holding on to more fluid than usual. The increased pressure in your leg vein and pressure from your growing baby adds on to the situation.

Swelling on legs, feet or ankle is normal but swelling on face and hands indicates a condition of preeclampsia and one must consult a doctor.

- Soak your feet in Epsom salt water for about 15-30 minutes. It is excellent naturopathy treatment.
- Excess salt in diet contributes a lot to swelling, replace it with sendha namak (rock salt).
- Massage works well in swollen feet (please refer chapter-5).
- Vipritkarni with wall support (yoga posture — please check chapter-3) helps alleviate the situation.
- Consume vitamin C and E rich food.
- Avoid long period of standing.
- Use cold compresses on swollen foot.

Bleeding or Spotting

A common complaint for pregnant women is spotting during first few months. Generally, this occurs near the date of your period cycle. You can try these suggested treatments as a quick measure, but it is also recommended to consult a doctor.

- Proper bedrest.
- Raise the footrest of your bed up by 30 cm (12 inches), or place a pillow under your thighs to raise the level of your legs then your body.
- Place a mud pack or cold wet towel on your lower abdomen.
- Drink rice water.

Once the bleeding stops, you must take complete bed rest for 4-5 days, and then, for the next 2-3 months when your period date is near, you take care by doing much less work and by resting well.

....

Here we conclude the chapter on caring for yourself and your fetus during pregnancy. This chapter is all about the vital care that needs to be taken by the mother during her pregnancy. Sonowlet'smovetooneofmyfavoritetopic– prenatal yoga, to learn the highly beneficial yoga postures during pregnancy.

Prenatal Yoga

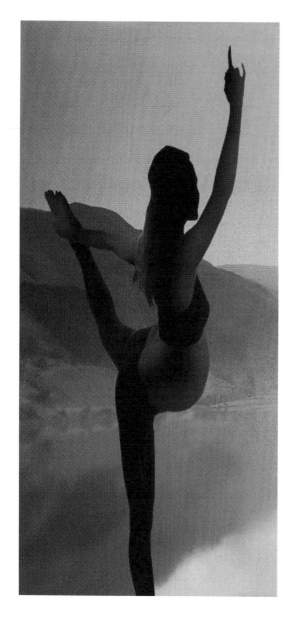

Earlier women did not need separate physical exercise as they were doing all household work by themselves like grinding, mopping, washing cloths and so on which keeps their body flexible, strong and energetic but today's scenario is changed and our modern lifestyle make our body less flexible, less energetic, weak and under-utilized. During pregnancy you highly require to have strong pelvic, abdominal, back, neck and thighs for smooth pregnancy and easy labor. You can adopt any form of exercise like walking, swimming, cycling, or yoga. Choose swimming or cycling if you are already doing it before pregnancy, instead of learning a new thing. So, prenatal yoga is the best thing that you can do for yourself and for your baby.

Benefits of yoga during pregnancy:

1   It gives you good stamina and strength.
2   Those who exercise consistently often sleep better and wake up feeling fresh.
3   Yoga calms your nervous system.
4   It causes your brain to release endorphins. It is a feel-good chemical that give you a naturally happy mood and reduce stress and anxiety.
5   An active body encourages active bowel.
6   Yoga's different postures helps to relieve pain from lower back, shoulder, hip and chest.
7   It helps to bring the fetus into a natural birth position.
8   During labor, the mother is able to control her body and mind and can loosen up muscles that facilitate labor.
9   During labor she can even push properly with trained and strong muscles.
10 It also helps her to recover faster post delivery.
11 *Pranayam* helps to improve lungs capacity and generate good flow of oxygen in body which is good not only for mother but also for the baby.

Caution:

- All *asanas* should be learned from a yoga therapist.
- Wear loose and comfortable clothes.
- Never over stretch your body, always go with your flexibility and strength.

In this chapter we will discuss different yoga postures for all trimesters, coupled with Pranayama, highly beneficial breathing exercises and some positions which would be beneficial during first stage of labor.

3.1 Yoga for the first trimester

In the first trimester, the fetus is not completely stable as the placenta is in developing stage, so in this period one should be more careful and we will target such exercises that are light and easy which also gives good workout to your muscles and generates good circulation in the body.

1 Sukshma vyayam

Sukshma vyayam is also known as joint stretching and rotation. This should be performed before starting any other *asanas*. This is very safe and easy form of exercise, and you can perform them throughout your pregnancy.

Perform Ankle stretch for 10 counts. Also perform all rotations for 10 counts, clockwise and anticlockwise.

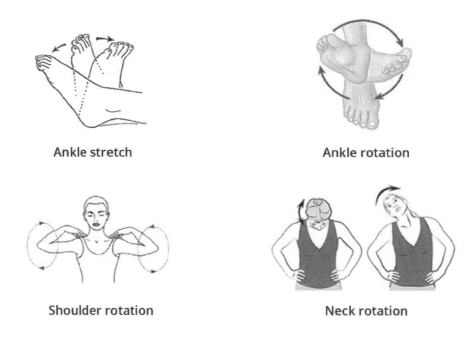

Ankle stretch

Ankle rotation

Shoulder rotation

Neck rotation

Figure 1

Benefits

- They prepare your body to perform other asanas.
- They remove blocks and clips in muscles, and strengthen them.
- They increase flexibility of ligaments.
- They relax the body and generate a good energy flow.

2 Leg raising

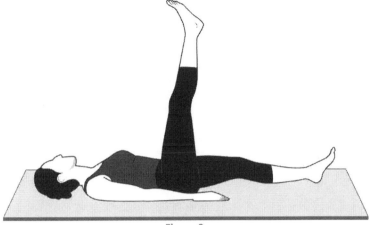

Figure 2

- Lie down on your back
- Place hands near to your body
- Slowly raise your right leg up to 90° degree without bending your knee and with exhalation slowly drop your right leg. Repeat the procedure 10 times.
- Repeat the same procedure with your left leg.

Caution:

- Do not raise your leg more than 90° as it puts pressure on your belly in the later stages of your pregnancy.
- After 6 months you may also bend your left knee and may raise your right leg for better support - and vice versa.

Benefits:

- Strengthens hamstring and pelvic muscles.
- Tones legs and improves flexibility.
- Generates good circulation in legs, pelvic area and in lower back.

3 Hip lift

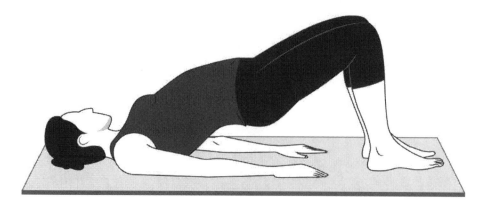

Figure 3

- Lie on your back with your arms on your sides, knees bent and feet on the floor apart in line of your hip.
- Lift your hips toward the ceiling.
- Hold the posture for 5-10 seconds and come down.
- Repeat for 7-10 rounds.

Benefits:

- Works on hips, abs and back muscles.
- Relaxes your lower back and relieves pain.

4 Spinal twist

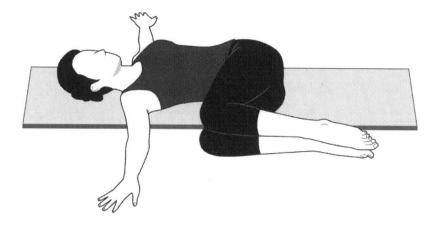

Figure 4

- Lie down on your back.
- Keep your hands on level with your shoulders.
- Bend your knees, keep your feet together and bring them towards your hip.
- Slowly twist your body to the right side and move your face towards left side.
- Hold the stretch for 5 deep and slow breathing.
- Repeat the same procedure with the other side.
- Repeat three times.

Benefits:

- Relieves pain from lower back and strengthens lower back muscles

5 Cat-cow posture

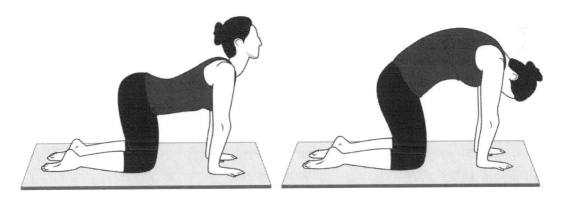

Figure 5

- Assume a four legged position.
- Make sure your palms, knees and feet are in a straight line.
- As you inhale, bend your spine in a concave shape and look up and slightly expand your belly – the cow posture.
- As you exhale, arch your spine in a convex shape, drop your head so your chin rests on your sternum notch and very slightly contract your belly – the cat posture.
- Repeat slowly and rhythmically 5-7 times.

Benefits:

- Relaxes spine and back muscles.
- Releases back pain and discomfort in back.

- Improves blood circulation in back.

6 Vakarasan

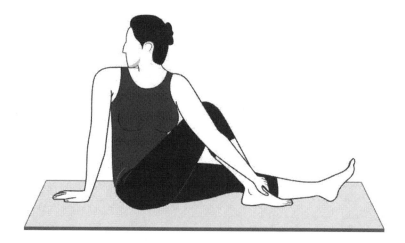

Figure 6

- Assume a sitting position with your legs stretched in front of you.
- Bend your right leg and place your right foot in line with your left knee.
- Cross your left hand to your right side and try to hold your right ankle with your left palm.
- Place your right hand back beside your spine and move your head so it is in line with your right shoulder.
- Hold this position for 15 to 30 seconds. And then slowly come back by releasing your left hand and then your right hand.
- Repeat for the other side.

Benefits:

- Improves flexibility in the lower region.
- Is good for the lower back and tailbone.
- Works well for your liver.

7 Matsyasana

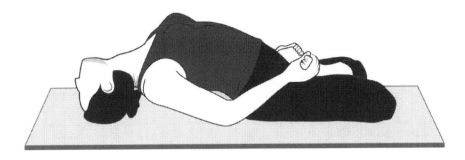

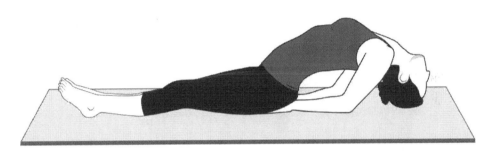

Figure 7

- Lie down on your back.
- Fold your left leg, then your right leg and make *padmasana* (Lotus pose)
- With the support of your palms on the floor, lift your head and place your crown on the ground.
- After getting better balance, release your palms and hold your toes with your figures. Make sure your elbows are bent and touching the ground.
- Divide your body weight between your head and elbows.
- Hold this posture for 15-30 seconds
- Come back slowly by straightening your head first with the support of your palms and then release the *padmasana*.

Caution:

- If you can't hold your toes, then don't force yourself. Place your palms on your belly by resting your elbow firmly on the floor.
- If making *padmasana* is difficult please don't force yourself rather opt for the easy version shown in the second image to gain all the benefits of asana.

Benefits:

- Stimulates thyroid and parathyroid glands.
- Stimulates pituitary gland.
- Strengthens legs and chest region.

8 Baddha konasana with Ashwini mudra

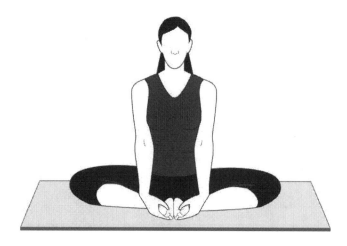

Figure 8

- Sit with your legs straight out in front of you.
- Bend your knees and pull your feet towards your pelvis as close as you can, with soles of your feet touching each other.
- Drop your knees towards the floor and pull your feet inside as shown in figure.
- With your index, middle finger and thumb grab toes of each foot.
- Contract your perineum (or vaginal muscles) for 5-7 seconds and release. (ashwini mudra / kegel exercise)
- Repeat these contractions 15-30 times, and at the end release the posture.

Benefits:

- Strengthens your pelvic floor, hamstring and lower back muscles.
- Helps constipation and hemorrhoids.
- Makes birth canal flexible and strong.

9 Ardh-ustrasana

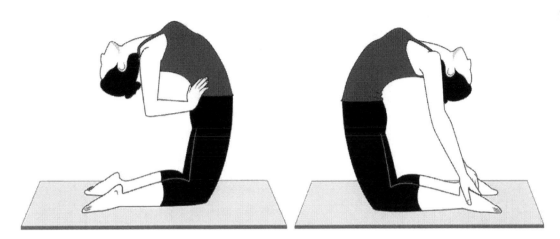

Figure 9

- Sit in vajrasana (kneeling and sitting on your heels)
- Come up on your knees.
- Spread your knees slightly apart just under your hips, and arrange your feet in the straight line with your knees.
- Place your palms on your waist and bend backward gently as far as you can.
- Now slowly reach down to hold your left foot with your left palm, and right foot with your right palm.
- Hold this posture for 15-30 seconds then slowly and smoothly come back to *vajrasana*.
- If you cannot perform the final posture due to less flexibility please do not force yourself. You can perform an easy level as shown in image one (just keeping your hand on your waist and backward bend), gradually when flexibility increases you can reach to the final posture.

Benefits:

- Stretches uterine muscles and lower abs (abdominal muscles), bringing them good blood circulation.
- Strengthens uterus, back and spine.

10 Tadashan

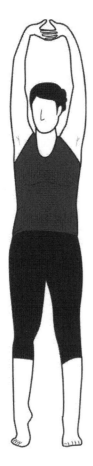

Figure 10

- Stand erect with legs slightly apart with the hands by your sides.
- Raise both hands above your head, lift your feet and look straight ahead.
- Interlock the fingers and turn hands upwards. Adjust your gaze straight to the horizontal level.
- Hold this posture for 30 seconds.

Benefits:

- Strengthens leg muscles, knees and ankles.
- Generates good balance in your body.
- Gives a good stretch to whole body.

11 Belly rotation

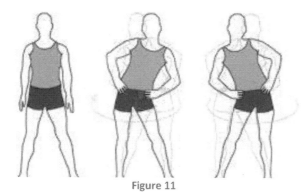

Figure 11

- Stand with your feet apart and palms on your waist.
- Rotate your belly making circles clockwise and anticlockwise.
- Repeat 10 times in both directions.

Benefits:

- Removes lower back pain and generates good blood circulation in the lower part of the body.

12 Trikonasana

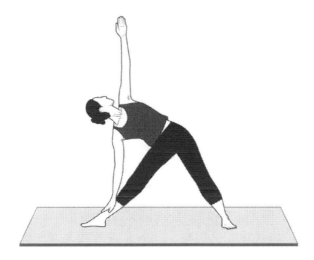

Figure 12

- Assume a standing posture, with your feet about 1 meter apart.
- Stretch your arms out at shoulder level, palms facing the ground.
- Exhale and bend your left side, till your left hand rests on your ankle, and your right hand goes straight up.
- Look up at the tips of your fingers.
- Hold this position for 10-30 second and slowly come back.
- Repeat with the other side

Benefits:

- Strengthens the side part of your back.
- Relieves back pain.

13 Ardha chakarasan

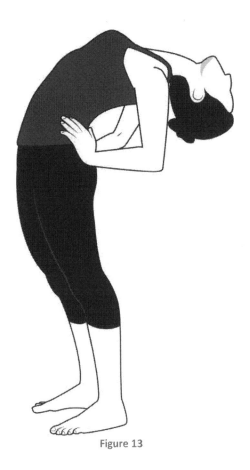

- Assume a standing position, and place your palms on the back side of your waist.
- Inhale and slowly bend backwards as far as you can, but be gentle and keep your eyes open.
- Hold this posture for 10-20 seconds and slowly come back.

Benefits:

- Gives a good stretch to your belly.
- Relieves backache or any discomfort.

Figure 13

3.2 Yoga for the Second Trimester

In the second trimester, the placenta is now fully developed and your pregnancy is more stable. You can perform maximum *asanas* in this trimester as the chances of miscarriage are negligible compared to the first trimester, and your belly has not -

grown as much as it does in the third trimester, so performing asanas does not discomfort your body as it does in last trimester. As a result, this is the best time to perform varieties of *asanas*.

In this trimester you will be working on strengthening, stabilizing your body, especially on your pelvic floor, glutes (gluteus muscles) and legs.

Following are some new posture which can be started in the second trimester along with a few postures given in first trimester. Check the sequence of postures to be performed, given in the table at the end of the topic.

1 Leg raising with modification

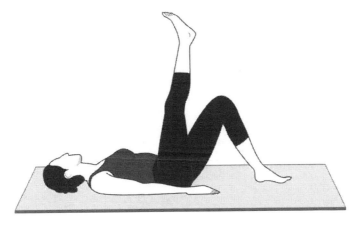

Figure 14

- Lie down on your back
- Place hands near to your body
- Bend your left leg to rest the foot on the floor for support.
- Inhale and slowly raise your right leg up to 90⁰ degree without bending your knee.
- Exhale slowly as you drop your right leg.
- Repeat 10 times.
- Repeat the same procedure with the other leg.

Benefits:

- Strengthens hamstring muscles and pelvic muscles.
- Tones legs and improves flexibility.
- Generates good circulation in legs, pelvic area and in lower back.

2   Cat-Cow posture – with modification

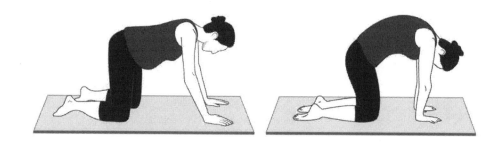

Figure 15

- In the second trimester when you inhale, don't make the cow posture. Means keep your spine straight instead of doing a concave arch. When you exhale, you can drop your head and make a convex arch of your spine (cat posture, as before).
- Repeat for 5-7 rounds.

3 Cat-Cow posture with belly rotation

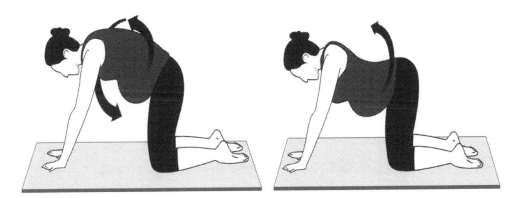

Figure 16

- Assume a four legged position on the floor.
- Rotate your belly and hips to make good big circles clockwise, and then anticlockwise.
- Make 5-7 circles each way.

Benefits:

- Relieves back pain and loosens up tight pelvis.
- Generates flexibility and good circulation in the belly, back and pelvic area.
- Relaxes muscles of the pelvic floor and back.

4 Cat-Cow with leg kick

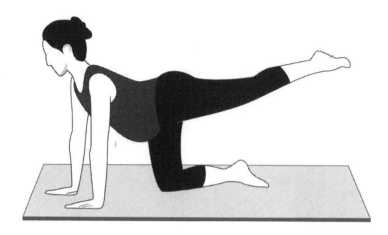

Figure 17

- Assume a four legged position on the floor.
- Lift your left leg backwards and slightly upwards without jerk, and then slowly return it to the floor.
- Make 10 lifts with each leg.

Benefits:

- Strengthens legs, gluts, pelvic floor and back.
- Helps leg pain and back pain.

5 Cat-Cow with knee lift

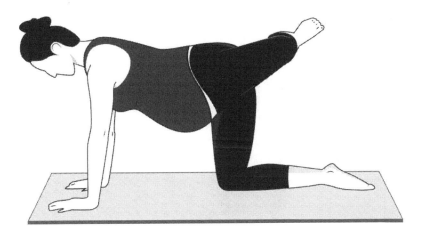

Figure 18

- Assume a four legged position on the floor.
- Slowly lift your left knee as far as possible to your left side, and hold for 3 seconds.
- Return to the floor.
- Make 10 lifts with each leg.

Benefits:

- Open up pelvic muscles and makes them strong.
- Helps relieve back pain.

6 Viparit karni with wall support

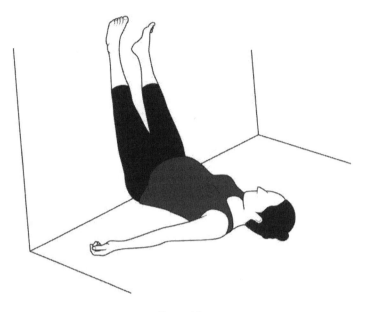

Figure 19

- Lie on the floor, with your legs raised, knees straight but not very tight, feet against the wall, and buttocks 30-40 cm away from the wall.
- Keep your thighs away from your abdomen, so you don't block blood circulation in your groin region.
- Ensure your back, neck and head are in a straight line, with your chin slightly lowered to avoid arching your neck and tightening your cervical vertebrae.
- Keep your arms at a slight distance from your trunk, if possible with your palms turned upwards, thus resting your shoulder blades properly on the ground.
- Hold for 30 seconds to 2 minutes.

Benefits:

- Is very beneficial to people with a hollowed chest and stooping shoulders.
- Refreshes your back and legs.
- Relieves varicose veins, and helps decongest swollen ankles and feet.
- To remedy an overly arched back, press your lumbar region against the ground as well, a movement helped by the raised position of your feet.

7   Half squats

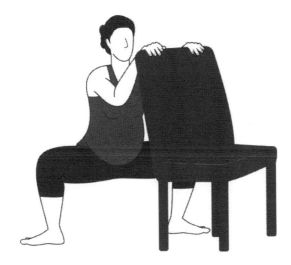

Figure 20

- Stand alongside a chair, keeping your back straight and upright.
- Bend gently from the knees and hips and slowly lower down yourself. Go only half way to the ground.
- Use the chair for balance only. Do not put any body weight on it. Keep looking forward and resist the temptation to bend your back.
- Hold this position for 3 second and slowly come back.
- Repeat for 5-7 rounds.

Benefits:

- Strengthens pelvic floor, legs, thighs and hamstring muscles.
- Helps your fetus to come into the right position.
- Helps lower back pain.

8 Veer Bhadarasana

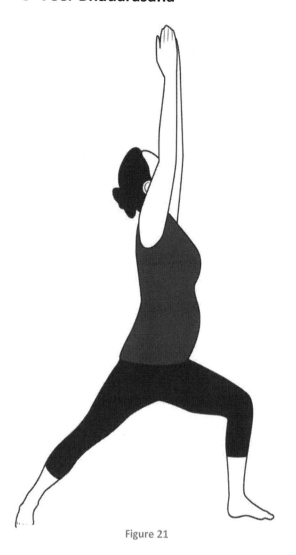

Figure 21

- Stand in Tadasana (legs together, toes touching, back straight and neck aligned with the spine).
- Inhaling, step 1 metre out.
- Exhaling, turn your right foot out to 90° and left foot slightly inwards.
- Inhale; then as you exhale, bend the right knee so that it is in line with your toes, with your thighs parallel to the mat. Keep your left leg straight and strong.
- Your face, chest, hips and right knee should be facing in the same direction as the right foot.
- Drop the hips as much as you can without moving the knee over the ankle.
- Tuck the tailbone inwards and make sure that your torso is aligned above the hipbones so that you are not tilted forward.

- Inhaling, lift your arms above the head and make the namskar mudra. Stretch your fingers towards the sky. Feel the stretch along your back leg, across your stomach and upwards from your chest.
- Keep your head in a neutral position, gazing forward. Hold the posture for 15-30 seconds.
- To release the posture, inhale, press the back heel firmly into the floor and reach up through the arms, straightening the right knee. Turn the feet forward and release the arms with an exhalation.
- Take a few breaths, then turn the feet to the left and repeat for the same time.
- Return to *Tadasana* (standing position), when you're finished.

Benefits:

- Expands the chest fully allowing for full and deeper breaths.
- Cures stiffness in neck, shoulders and back.
- Stretches chest, lungs, shoulders, neck and belly.
- Strengthens shoulders, arms and muscles of the back.
- Strengthens and stretches thighs, calves and ankles.
- Reduces pain in the knees, back, tailbone and from the legs.

Table for sequence of postures in second trimester

1	Sukshma vyayam	9	Baddhakonasan with Ashwini mudra
2	Leg raising with modification	10	Tadasana
3	Hip lift	11	Trikonasana
4	Spinal twist	12	Belly rotation
5	Cat-cow posture with modification	13	Ardha chakarasana
6	Cat-cow with belly rotation	14	Viparit karani with wall support
7	Cat-cow with leg kick	15	Veer bhadrasana
8	Cat-cow with knee lift	16	Half squats

3.3 Yoga for the Third Trimester

During third trimester of your pregnancy you should focus on *asanas* that open your hip, thereby helping your body to prepare for delivery.

You can continue all *asanas* from the second trimester, but in Ardha chakarasana take a very little arch of your back. You can start the asanas below from 7 and a half months.

1 Full squat

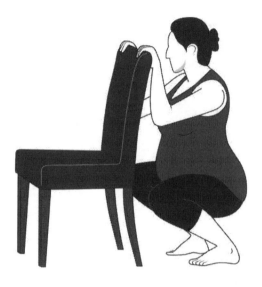

Figure 22

- Take a firm hold of a window grill or back of the chair with your legs about 2 feet apart.
- Bend your knees, lower your tailbone slowly, keeping your feet flat and firm on the floor.
- Hold this position for 5 seconds and come back slowly without a jerk.
- Repeat this for 5-10 counts twice a day.

Benefits:

- Strengthens pelvic floor, legs, thighs and hamstring muscles.
- Helps your baby to get into the right position.
- Helps lower back pain.
- Opens up pelvic area

2 Kali asana

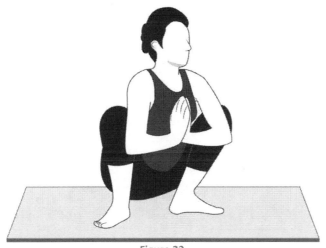

Figure 23

- Stand straight with legs about 2 feet apart, keeping some support to your back side.
- Bend your knees slowly and lower your hips near to the floor, keeping your feet flat and firm on the floor, with back support.
- Make the *namaskar mudra* in between your both knees.
- Hold the posture for 15-30 seconds twice a day, then slowly come back without a jerk.

Benefits:

- Strengthens legs, thighs, back, pelvic floor, ankle and knee.
- It's a great pelvic opener.
- Corrects baby's position in the womb.

3 Butterfly

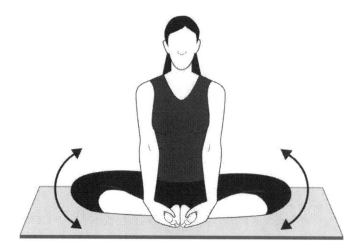

Figure 24

- Sit in sukhasana (cross-legged position)
- Bring the feet as close together as possible to the groin. Hold your feet with your palms.
- Slowly and steadily move both knees up and down as far as possible, like the wings of a butterfly. Make the movement smoothly, without forcing yourself.
- Continue moving your legs for 60-90 seconds.

Benefits:

- Strengthens muscles of thighs, legs and pelvis, which is good for labor.
- Facilitates the contraction-expansion capacity of buttocks and pelvic muscles.

4   Grinding exercise

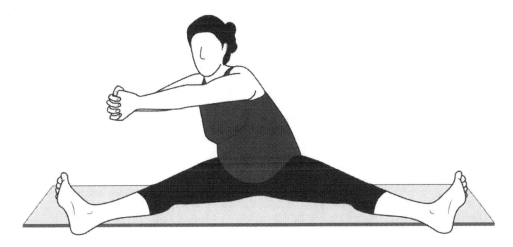

Figure 25

- Sit on the floor with your back straight and legs spread apart in front of you.
- Clasp your hands and outstretch your arms at shoulder height in front of you.
- Move your torso from right to left, slightly coming forward but not to a level which puts pressure on your upper abdominal region. Don't bend backwards.
- Make 7-10 rotations clockwise and then anticlockwise.

Benefits:

- Strengthens pelvic floor, thighs and abdominal muscles.
- Initiates baby movement.
- Relieves back pain and tightness in hamstrings, and opens up hip joint.

Table for sequence of postures in third trimester

1 Sukshma vyayam	11 Grinding exercise
2 Leg raising with modification	12 Tadasana
3 Hip lift	13 Trikonasana
4 Spinal twist	14 Belly rotation

67

5 Cat-cow posture with modification	15 Ardha chakarasana
6 Cat-cow with belly rotation	16 Viparit karani with wall support
7 Cat-cow with leg kick	17 Veer bhadrasana
8 Cat-cow with knee lift	18 Half squats
9 Baddhakonasan with Ashwini mudra	19 Full squats
10 Butterfly	20 Kali asana

3.4 Pranayama and some other breathing exercises

Pranayama is the art of yogic breathing or controlled breathing, a scientific breathing practice that has lots of benefits not only for your body but also for your mind and spirit.

Pranayama is a Sanskrit word which literally translates into "extension of the *prana* or breath", where *prana* means life-force or vital energy that pervades the body, and *ayama* means to extend or draw out the breath. *Prana* is the link between mind and consciousness, and its physical manifestation is breath.

Your breath has a direct connection with your mind so by practicing pranayama you can actually influence your mind, and bring about calm and peace and a deep relaxed state of body and mind. According to Hatha Yoga Pradipika, "When breath wanders, the mind is unsteady, and when breath is still, so is the mind."

Pranayama is the part of the yoga system that teaches you the art of extending your breath in many different ways. When practicing it your breath needs to be skillfully inhaled, exhaled and retained. It teaches you to change the depth, rate and pattern of breathing.

Breathing is vital for our survival as it is the only way we can send oxygen into our body and into our organs. We can live for months without consuming food and days without water, however we can only survive a few minutes without breathing. Learning the breathing techniques will positively affect your actions and thoughts. Every thought you have changes the rhythm of your breath. When you are happy your breathing is rhythmic, and when you are stressed it is irregular and interrupted. Mastering the art of breathing is a crucial step towards self-healing and survival.

Pranayama focuses on the conscious inhalation of oxygen and exhalation of carbon dioxide. It ensures that adequate oxygen flows through your body. This is most crucial during pregnancy, when your unborn baby completely depends on you for its supply of oxygen. Having the correct balance of oxygen and carbon dioxide through conscious breathing makes your lungs stronger, and makes your blood pure. Obviously, this helps the healthy functioning of your body so that you can take optimum care of your baby.

Benefits of Pranayama

In general …

- Pranayama techniques are beneficial in treating a range of stress related disorders.
- Pranayama improves autonomic functions (like blood pressure, heart and breathing rates, body temperature digestion and metabolism).
- Pranayama helps relieve the symptoms of asthma.
- Pranayama reduces the signs of oxidative stress in the body.
- Pranayama causes changes in the cardio-respiratory system including lowering of blood pressure – shown by a number of studies.
- Certain pranayama are excellent for weight loss.
- Pranayama increases the flow of oxygen in the body and removes carbon dioxide, which helps to detoxify your internal system.
- Pranayama practiced every day assists a steady mind, strong will power and sound judgement.
- Pranayama practiced regularly can extend life and enhance your perception of life.

And in pregnancy …

- Pranayama during pregnancy is known to release positive hormones, which eliminates negative thoughts and brings the mind to a calm and relaxed state, which is very important for the expectant mother and her unborn child.
- Pranayama makes the expectant mother conscious of controlled breathing, which is proven to aid in a normal delivery as she has learned how to control her breathing.
- Pranayama increases the flow of oxygen, which in turn increases the blood circulation throughout the mother's and unborn child's bodies.

- Pranayama sessions help in removing toxins from both mother and unborn child.

1. Anulom-vilom pranayam (Alternate nostril breathing)

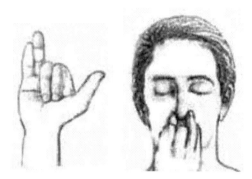

- Sit in any comfortable asana, such as *padmasana*, *vajrasana* or *sukhasana* (cross legs).
- Make the mudra shown in the picture with your right hand.
- Close the right nostril with your right hand thumb, and breathe in slowly and fully through the left nostril; and then exhale from your right nostril; and then inhale again from your right nostril and finally exhale from your left nostril. This completes one round.
- Continue with any number of rounds, the minimum being 7-11 rounds, and there being no maximum.
- Breathe deeply and slowly at all times.

Benefits:

- Balances and calms our nervous system thus relaxing the mind, and removing stress.
- Strengthens respiratory system by increasing lungs capacity to inhale and retain air.
- Enriches the blood with oxygen, which is then beneficial for the brain, lungs, heart, and capillaries.
- Cleanses 72,000 *nadis* (channels in the body), according to yoga science.

70

- Creates a wonderful sense of peace and blissfulness, as if you were moved into a new world.

2 Sheetali prayanama

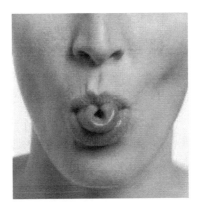

- Sit in a comfortable meditative posture.
- Protrude your tongue from the mouth and extend it to a comfortable distance.
- Roll the sides up so that it forms a tube.
- Breathe in slowly and deeply through the tube like tongue.
- Close your mouth, at the end of inhalation and try to gulp air accumulated in your mouth once, then hold your breath upto your normal capacity .
- Exhale from your nose, whenever you want.

Benefits:

- Cools the stomach, liver and whole body, as this is a cooling *pranayama*.
- Helps in high blood pressure and acidity.
- Purifies blood and improves digestion.

3 Four stage breathing

Assume a comfortable position either sitting or lying down. Relax your body and let your mind be peaceful.

(1) Abdominal breathing
- Concentrate on your abdomen.
- Let your belly rise as you inhale, and then fall as you exhale.
- Breathe deeply and slowly.
- Repeat for 5 rounds.

Benefits:

- Activates abdominal and lower back muscles, and relieves pain if any. This is important as it is very necessary to keep the abs and back flexible for normal and easy labor.

(2) Thoracic breathing
- Concentrate on your chest.
- Let your chest expand as you inhale and feel contraction in the same area as you exhale.
- Repeat for 5 rounds.

Benefits:

- Develops full capacity of lungs which is very vital for active and easy labor.
- Generally, after the fifth or sixth month, because of her growing belly, the mother-to-be feels ineffective and effortful in breathing. Hence, this exercise improves such difficulties, and generates good oxygen levels in the body.

(3) Clavicle breathing
- Inhale deeply, pulling your shoulders slightly back and filling more air into your upper clavicles, and allow your shoulders to return to their normal position as you exhale slowly.
- Repeat for 5 rounds.

Benefits:

- Works on the upper part of your lungs and improves its capacity.
- This breathing helps to relax and distressed mother-to-be, and also brings amazing peace.

(4) All three together

- Inhale slowly and deeply and fill your abdomen, then expand your lungs and lastly bring your shoulder back and hold this position for few seconds.
- Exhale slowly and deeply and allow your shoulders to return to their normal position, contract your chest and then contract your abdominal muscles.
- Repeat for 5 rounds.

Benefits:

- This is full yogic breathing and rejuvenates your entire body.

4 Om chanting

- Sit in a comfortable posture.
- Close your eyes and relax your body and mind. Concentrate on your *agna chakra* (third eye)
- Chant "OM" 5-7 times.

Benefits:

- Calms the mind and body, brings all positive energy.
- Enlightens both mother and baby.

3.5 Some postures to use during labor

The process of labor is divided into three stages. Please refer to Chapter 5 *All about Labor* if you want to find out more.

During stage 1A, it's always advisable to be mobile. Walking or doing household work during stage 1A aids your contractions, speeds up dilation of the cervix and helps your baby position itself properly in your womb.

During stage 1C, you may not be able to walk, but you can adopt one of the following upright positions, rather than just lying down. It would be a good idea to play with them during your pregnancy so you are familiar with them before your labor starts.

All these postures help to ease pain, speed up Stage 1C and encourage your baby to move deeper in your pelvis. As these are upright positions, gravity can also help your baby to be in the right position for birth. They also have the added advantage that they allow you to be massaged easily on your back, hips or thighs - wherever you wish pain to be eased.

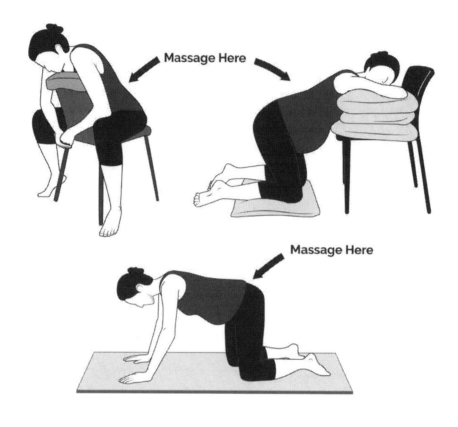

So it concludes the chapter on yoga and breathing exercises you can practice during your pregnancy to optimize the health of both baby in-utero and yourself, and also helps to manage any pain.

These exercises are vital for preparing your body and mind for the time when your baby will be born. They provide you with a wonderful means of maximizing your body's strength, flexibility, focus and endurance.

By the means of practicing these exercises, you will develop marvelously useful resources to use during your labor, so you can deliver your beloved baby as safely as possible, and have as close to an easy and pain-free labor as possible. You will then indeed bless the time you spent doing this prenatal yoga throughout the months of your pregnancy and make that miraculous day an ideal one!

WORLD OF MEDITATION

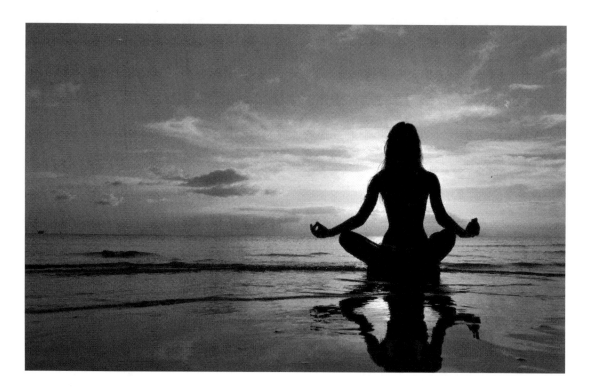

Pregnancy involves lots of hormonal changes which bring changes in both your physical and emotional states. Your baby continues to grow each passing week and it's so very pleasing to feel it taking shape right there inside you. At the same time, you are witnessing new developments within yourself – some wondrous, some interesting, and perhaps some difficult to handle. You may also feel a little anxious, stressed or experience disconcerting mood swings. Possibly, fear and common health complaints are afflicting your emotional state of mind.

What if you could happily accept all the changes that are happening and enjoy this extraordinary phase of your life to the maximum? Yes, this can be possible with a few minutes of sitting by yourself with your eyes closed in meditation.

Meditation is the best way to pamper yourself, relax and calm your body and mind.

Benefits of Meditation

- Connects you with your inner world
- Calms and composes you
- Balances your body, mind and soul
- Bonds you deeply with your baby
- Inculcate good values (*sanskar*) in your baby
- Feel better about your changing body
- Prepare yourself for birth and beyond
- Helps to increase the level of *prana* (life force energy)

In this chapter we will discuss a couple of meditations and therapies which are very easy to practice, at the same time make you feel relaxed and enlightened. Let's have a look into the fascinating spiritual world of meditation. You can see what is possible for you and choose the ones you prefer.

4.1 Chakra Meditation

The Sanskrit word Chakra literally translates to wheel or disk. In yoga, this term refers to wheels of energy throughout the body. There are seven main chakras, which align the spine, starting from the base of the spine through to the crown of the head. This invisible energy, called Prana, is a vital life force, which keeps you vibrant, healthy, and alive. Each of the seven main chakras contains bundles of nerves and regulates major organs as well as your psychological, emotional, and spiritual state of being. It is essential that these seven chakras stay open and aligned. If there is a blockage, energy cannot flow. Keeping a chakra open is a bit more of a challenge, but not so difficult when you have awareness.

Each *chakra* [energy center] has a special role in your body and mind, and just by focusing on it and chanting its specific mantra you can actually charge (or energize) it and acquire all its positive benefits.

For the Chakra Meditation specially prepared for pregnancy, we will focus in sequence on three of your *chakras*, firstly on your *Muladhar chakra* (Root chakra), then on your *swadhisthan chakra* (Sacral chakra) and finally on your *Agna chakra* (Third Eye chakra).

Chakra Meditation Process

Sit comfortably on the floor or middle of the bed (not on its edge) with crossed legs and use a pillow to support your back. Softly close your eyes and take 7-10 deep and slow breaths. Relax your body and calm your mind.

Muladhar chakra:

- Slowly focus on your *muladhar chakra* (Root chakra) which is located on the base of your spine, on your pelvic floor.
- Keeping your focus on the chakra, start to chant the mantra 'LAMM' (or 'LAM' which rhymes with 'sum '). Try to use a low pitch and feel vibration on the area of your muladhar chakra.
- Keep chanting for 3-5 minutes.

Benefits:

Just by focusing and chanting the LAMM mantra you can energize this chakra. The Root chakra is related to your excretory system, vagina and the cervix. It is related to stability and emotions like letting go of fear and feeling safe. Imbalance in this chakra creates anxiety disorders, fears or nightmares, urinary tract infection, constipation, lower back pain or leg pain.

Thus you are able to minimize these problems and attain a wholesome emotional state. It is important to have healthy and charged Root chakra for a smooth labor as the health of your vagina and cervix is closely related with this chakra.

Swadhisthan chakra:

- Now focus on your Swadhisthan chakra (Sacral chakra) located four fingers down below your naval.
- Chant 'VAMM' repeatedly with the same low pitch for 3-5 minutes, trying to feel vibration in the area of your Swadhisthan chakra.

Benefits:

This chakra is related with the reproductive system, kidneys, lower back, intestines and ability of creating a new soul within you. It is also the centre of feeling, emotion, pleasure, sensuality, intimacy and connection.

Energizing this chakra helps to create good energy flow around this chakra, and also deepens bonding with your little one. Well energized chakra also allows you to let go, to move on, and to feel change and transformation occurring within your body along with experiencing the present moment at its fullness. A well energized Swadhisthan chakra also reduces the chances of complications in labor and common problems during pregnancy.

Agna chakra

- Now focus on the Agna chakra (Third Eye chakra). It is located in between your eyebrows.
- Chant 'OM' with the same low pitch for 3-5 minutes, again trying to feel vibration in the area of your Agna chakra.

Benefits:

This chakra is related to your mind and soul. When it is energized, it brings you firmness, clarity, and spiritual up-lift. Thus this chakra gives you amazing feelings of deep satisfaction, calmness and enlightenment, a sense of deep silence and stillness. It also helps to balance your mind and body, as well as provides strength and confidence for your labor and beyond.

4.2 Aroma Meditation

In aromatherapy, essential oils, extracted from plants are inhaled and they can have a beneficial effect on the mind and body. Some are relaxing, while others are energizing. For this reason, aroma therapy works very effectively during pregnancy, and you can use an aroma during meditation, though it's best to wait until you are past your first trimester, before you start using any.

There are a couple of different ways you can use an essential oil for direct inhalation.

- You can add 3 drops of it to warm water and inhale the vapor.
- You can heat 1-2 drops of oil diluted in water in a fragrance burner.

Aroma Therapy Process for Meditation

To use the aroma of an essential oil during meditation:

- Heat 1-2 drops of your chosen oil diluted in water in a fragrance burner, and let the room fill with the aroma.
- Sit comfortably with a good back support, and gently close your eyes.
- Take deep and slow breaths. As you inhale slowly, assume you are inhaling all positive energies into you and when you exhale slowly, release all your negative emotions. These negative emotions could be anything like fear, anxiety, worry, anger, stress but work on the ones that you are experiencing.
- Let yourself feel calm and relaxed, without any expectations and without any future plans.
- Enjoy this lightness and deep feeling of silence.

Essential oils to use:

- Citrus oils like tangerine and *neroli* (from the bitter orange tree) will uplift your mood and lower your stress levels.
- Chamomile and lavender oil will relax you and deal with insomnia.
- Eucalyptus will help to clear a blocked nose and cold.

Caution

As there are few essential oils which should not be used during pregnancy, so always consult an aromatherapist if you want to use any oils other than the ones above.

4.3 Music Therapy

A new study has found that music therapy can reduce psychological stress among pregnant women, and that it works excellently on stress, anxiety, fear and depression. The music seems to act like a medicine for the mind keeping it calm and composed. Naturally, this can be advantageous during your pregnancy! You can use it to counterbalance any lonely times and disturbed moods you may have.

Healing music like mantras, instrumental music or *ragas* are also wonderful to use.

Ragas

Ragas are pieces of music based on particular scales and notes (*swar*) and are central to classical Indian music. Unlike western classical music, which can be listened at any time of day, ragas are created for specific seasons and times of day. There are many ragas that are capable of providing all the calmness, if they are listened to during their proper allotted time.

Ragas play a mighty role in providing a peaceful environment for a pregnant woman and for her baby. Women who listen to ragas or mantras give birth to a child with a sharp memory.

Ayurveda also suggests some instrumental music by *veena* and *sitar*. These are both large stringed instruments that are plucked and used in classical Indian music, and sound quite different from each other.

You can purchase CDs that contain suitable ragas and play them in your home or download some of the below mentioned ragas from the internet.

Some of the most common *ragas* are:

- Raga Darbari and Raga Kalyani: relaxes and dissolves tension
- Raga Bhairavi: acts as a medicine for certain diseases like T.B.
- Raga Shivaranjini: works as a memory booster
- Raga Bhupali: controls blood pressure
- Raga Yaaman: reduces stress

Mantras

Playing mantras at home provides excellent positive vibrations to both you and your unborn baby.

The Navkar mantra, the Gayatri mantra, and the Adi shakti mantra, OM chanting and so on have excellent impact. You may choose mantras based on your own religious beliefs and what appeals most to you.

4.4 Reiki

Reiki is one of the best alternative therapies. It is a very safe, pure and spiritual therapy in which the therapist channels energy into the client's body via touch to stimulate the natural healing processes. It is a non-invasive, gentle healing technique that works on body, mind and spirit. It helps to relax and calm your mind and body, rejuvenates whole system, accelerating healing and promoting both good health and a strong immune system.

Reiki energy creates a deep bond between you and your unborn baby and will increase the baby's health and well-being. When a mother-to-be receives Reiki her fetus receives it as well. You can have Reiki from a professional reiki healer, but for daily practice you can follow these steps which are very easy and safe and also have all the above mentioned benefits.

Reiki process

- Sit on the yoga mat or on the middle of a bed.
- Gently close your eyes and take 7-10 deep and slow breaths.
- Gently place your hand on your growing tummy and visualize a beautiful and pure white light coming from God and entering into your crown chakra.
- Feel your crown chakra getting filled with the white light, and experience its pure energy.
- After filling your crown chakra the white light travels down and reaches to your agna chakra (third eye chakra). Feel your agna chakra getting filled with the white light, and experience its pure energy.
- After filling your *agna* chakra the white light travels further down and reaches your *vishudhdhi chakra* (throat chakra) near your larynx. Feel your *vishudhdhi* chakra getting filled with the white light.
- After filling your *vishudhdhi chakra the light* goes further downwards to your *anahat chakra* (heart chakra). Feel your heart filled with positive and pure energy from God.
- After filling your heart chakra the white light spreads from both your sides and enters into your hands coming out from both palms. (Many spiritual women feel very strong energy coming out from their palms.)
- As you have placed your palms on your tummy, feel the energy being transmitted into your belly and deep into your baby. Feel your baby absorbing this divine energy.
- Feel the white light curing all disorders, charging your body and increasing the health of your fetus.

- Once you feel fully charged, start talking to your baby, telling her that you are so keen to welcome her, what dreams you have made for her up-bringing. You can even talk with her about the labor process, explaining that it is going to be easy for both of you. Just open your heart to your baby. During reiki many women feel that their baby moves more and even turns towards their hands.
- After a good talk, happily say good-bye for now, but explain that you are always with her, and then slowly let the white light dissolve into your belly and after a deep breath slowly open your eyes.

···

So this now concludes the chapter on meditation. There is a lot for you to explore here! And then you'll need to decide which aspects of it you will use and how you'll incorporate them into your daily life.

Whichever practices you use, the end result is that you will be forging a closer relationship with your unborn baby and doing so in ways that are calming, nurturing and protective for both of you.

Both of you will settle more fully into the process that is pregnancy, thus maximizing the potential benefits it can provide. And this, of course, creates the strongest foundation for the future lives of both of you.

In the next chapter, we turn to the subject of acupressure, in which you'll learn how to use this therapy during your pregnancy to deal safely and effectively with any common health issues you may have, and also how to get benefited during your labor so that it progresses nicely.

All about Acupressure in Pregnancy

Acupressure is one of the best and most ancient alternate therapy for treating various diseases. It is such a wonderful science that just by putting pressure on a particular point in your body you can do healing. In this chapter we will discuss how acupressure helps before pregnancy, during labor, after pregnancy and also helps the baby.

Acupressure is beneficial because it:

- Boosts the health of the reproductive system.
- Solves almost all menstrual problems.
- Boosts hormones level.
- Leads to the proper growth of the baby during pregnancy.
- Reduces the chances of miscarriage.
- Reduces the chances of passing hereditary diseases to the child.
- Increases the chance of conceiving quickly.

How to give pressure

You can use your thumb or a wooden stick (jimmy) to pressure a point.	
Points located on your wrist joint should be pressurized with the thumb only. (You can even apply oil or a jelly-like substance to deeply massage the wrist points.)	

- The points on the wrist joint are situated a little deeper in the skin so pressure should be given with a little more deep effort.
- The stimulation speed should be slow not only for the wrist point but for all points, so for example, press the point for 4-5 seconds, release the pressure for 1-2 seconds, and press again ... and so on.
- The pressure for any points, wrist or otherwise, should be neither too strong nor too light. It should be deep and felt properly. On a hard hand it should be a little heavy, and on a soft hand it should be a little light.

- Duration: In hands reflexes, 1-2 minutes thrice a day per point is sufficient. In feet reflexes, 5 minutes thrice a day per point is sufficient.

Note:

- Remember that if you feel pain in point, it means the related organ is disturbed. As soon as you are cured, there won't be any pain in that point.
- Acupressure is very safe and gentle therapy with no side effects at all.
- During pregnancy, there are some acupressure points which should not be treated, so don't try any other points other than the ones given in this book or, if you wish, please consult a qualified acupressure therapist.

This chapter covers acupressure treatment for all stages of pre and post pregnancy as well as for the baby.

5.1 Acupressure for preparing for pregnancy

Points for hormonal imbalance

Following points are excellent to stimulate for curing hormonal imbalance and at the same time rejuvenates the hormonal levels in the body.

Pituitary gland points The pituitary gland points are located on the center of the thumb and the big toe. You should stimulate them twice or thrice a day for 1-2 minutes on your thumb and 3-4 minutes on your toe.	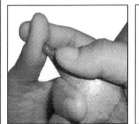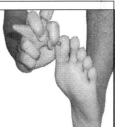

Thyroid point

The thyroid gland point is located just below your thumb on the mountain on both hands. You should stimulate this region twice or thrice a day for 2-3 minutes. This point is also very helpful for hypothyroidism (abnormally low activity of the thyroid) and obesity.

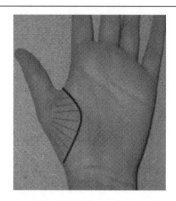

Adrenal gland point

The adrenal gland point is located on the palm of both hands between the index and middle fingers, between two metacarpals (finger bones). You should stimulate this point twice or thrice a day for 2-3 minute. This point is also excellent for reducing stress and depression.

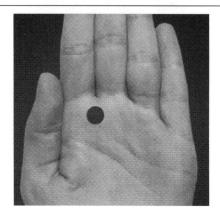

Points for blocked fallopian tubes

You can find this point right on your ankle joint. You should stimulate this point with your thumb or your fingers in a deep massaging movement for 2-3 minutes twice or thrice a day for better results.

This is an excellent point for fallopian tubes, and research shows that this point can also open up a blocked fallopian tube.

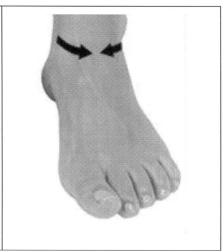

Points for scanty or painful period or white discharge

This point (rather region of points) is located on both sides of the wrist joint on both hands, just below the crease of the wrist joint and the area is about 3 fingers long. These are the points for your reproductive organs, and are excellent points for rejuvenating your whole reproductive system, as well as curing scanty or painful periods and the problem of white discharge. You should stimulate these points 4-5 minutes twice a day on each side. Use your thumb to pressure the point in a massaging movement.

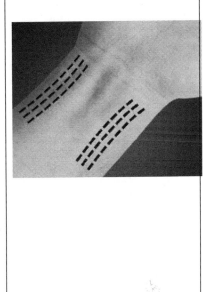

Any period problem may also occur because of hormonal imbalance, so you should also stimulate all the hormonal imbalance points for a better result.

Points to improve fertility

These points are excellent for improving your fertility. It is recommended that for the best results both partners should start stimulating them at least 2 months before planning to conceive. They stimulate your hormonal glands and lead it to their optimal levels, and also rejuvenate all reproductive organs. Both you and your partner should start stimulating these points for the healthy baby. It also minimizes the chance of hereditary diseases being passed to the baby and ensures a healthy pregnancy.

One should stimulate each point on both hands for 2-3 minutes twice a day.

(It is recommended to treat these points in spite of not having any problem, as these work as the best tonic for the whole reproductive system and hormones)

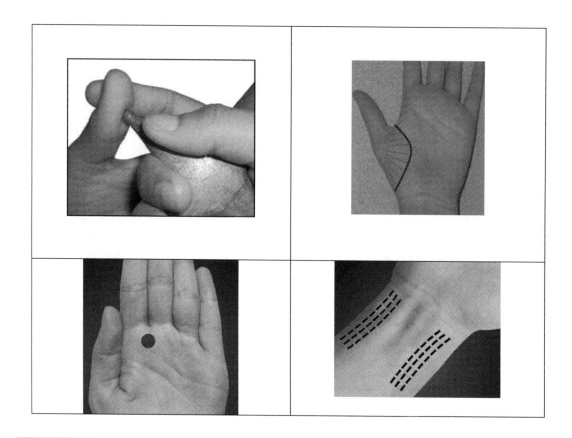

Points for high-blood pressure

K1

You can find this point in the center of the ball of your foot. It's always better to treat any high blood pressure before you conceive so you have better health during your pregnancy.

If your systolic pressure (the maximum pressure in the arteries) ranges between 167-180 mm Hg, you can stimulate this point for 1-2 minutes once a day. If it is still higher in the range of 190-200 mm Hg, you can stimulate the point 1-2 minute twice a day.

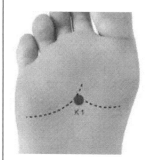

Note: Keep in mind that when doing this point you should be actively measuring your blood pressure every 2-3 days to keep a watch on your pressure, as this point is very powerful in decreasing the pressure. As soon as you start benefiting by having a normal or near to normal range of blood pressure, reduce the stimulation time gradually, and once you are within the normal range, stimulate this point for 1 minute once a day to maintain it.

Caution: You should not use this point during pregnancy.

Point for Constipation

This point (bearded area) is located on your chin. You can stimulate it with the help of your index finger or with your thumb. Stimulate this point for a minimum of 10 minutes and a maximum of 30-40 minutes for the best result.

This is a very safe point and also can be used during pregnancy for constipation.

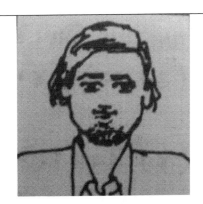

Point for Thyroid Dysfunction

This point is located on both hands, and for the best result you should stimulate each one for 5-10 minutes twice a day.

It is always better to treat thyroid dysfunction before pregnancy if any. One can also treat this point during pregnancy after consulting a good acupressure therapist.

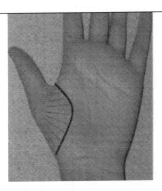

Points for Anemia

Anemia is a condition that should be treated before you conceive, because as a mother-to-be you require an optimal hemoglobin level for your and your baby's health. The range of hemoglobin level must be 11-12 g/dl during pregnancy (Please check Chapter 7 to find out what modern science says about this). Following are a set of points to increase hemoglobin level.

<table>
<tr>
<td>

SP10

When the knee is flexed (bent) this point is located on the inner side of the leg, 2 thumb-widths above the medial tip of the upper border of patella (kneecap).

Stimulate or press this point on both legs, one by one, in the press-and-release manner for 1 to 2 minutes with your thumb.

</td>
<td>

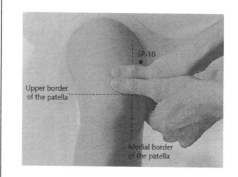

</td>
</tr>
<tr>
<td>

LIV8

When the knee is flexed this point is at the medial end inside of the leg of the popliteal crease (the crease under the knee). This point tones the blood and liver, and clears any excess heat.

Press these points on both legs for 1 to 2 minutes to get relief from anemia.

</td>
<td>

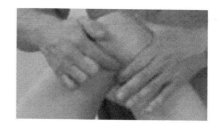

</td>
</tr>
<tr>
<td>

ST36

This point is located below the kneecap, 4 fingers width from the depression of the knee. It is called the 'tonification' point, as it tones both blood and body, as well as improving digestion and ability to absorb nutrients.

Press this point for 2-3 minutes every day for the absorption of iron and cure anemia.

</td>
<td>

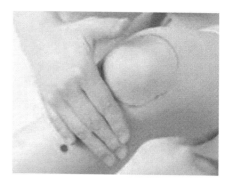

</td>
</tr>
</table>

5.2 Points to use during pregnancy

These points are useful for several common complaints of pregnancy – nausea and morning sickness, headache and constipation.

Points for Constipation

SJ6 You can find this point four finger width up from the wrist crease in the center of the arm. Press this point firmly for 3-5 minutes daily to help move the bowels. It helps to moisten the stool.	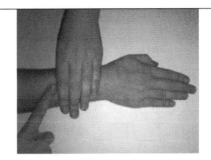
This point is located on your chin. You can stimulate it with the help of your index finger or with your thumb. Stimulate this point for a minimum of 10 minutes and a maximum of 30-40 minutes for the best result. This is a very safe point and also can be used during pregnancy for constipation.	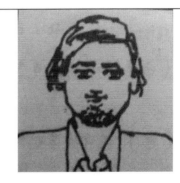

Point for Nausea and Morning Sickness

PC6 This point is three finger width above the transverse crease on your inner wrist. It lies directly between the two tendons you can feel there. Place firm pressure on this point for approximately five minutes every two hours, or whenever you feel nauseous.	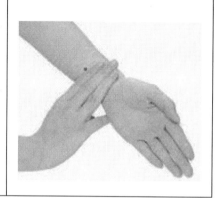

Points for Swollen Feet.

There is a sequence of reflex areas on your feet to stimulate for dealing with swollen feet. Once you have done this on one foot, you can then carry out the sequence on the other foot too.

Step 1 Walk your thumb through the reflex area for the lymph gland to encourage lymph drainage.	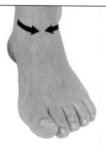
Step 2 Stimulate the reflex area for the kidneys to encourage the elimination of waste fluids.	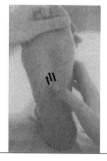

Step 3 Fingers walk down the reflex area for the upper chest area to encourage the drainage of the upper lymph drainage.	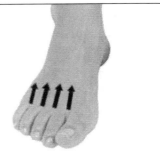

Point for Gestational diabetes

Gestational diabetes is the type of diabetes that's first diagnosed during pregnancy. Like the other types, gestational diabetes causes blood sugar levels to become too high.

Pancreas Point You can find this point on the palm of both hands between the ring and small fingers, between two metacarpals (finger bones). You should stimulate this point twice or thrice a day for 2-3 minute. This point works best to correct sugar level in the blood.	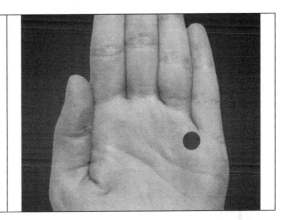

5.3   Points to use during labor

When a woman completes nine months of pregnancy, labor begins, and ideally within a few hours she gives birth to the baby. But sometimes the child-birth process takes a long time, and becomes unbearable. These acupressure points are most helpful for starting your labor naturally, to increase your contractions if they are mild, and making the child birth process faster, easier and safer.

Points for Speeding up Labor

Note of Caution:

These are very powerful points.

- Don't use them at any time during your pregnancy as they can induce premature labor.
- Use them only during your labor, i.e. only after the labor pains have truly begun. Please refer to the discussion about true and false labor pains in the section, Signs that Labor Has Begun, in Chapter 6 – All About Labor.
- If you are overdue then you can make use of them under the guidance of an acupressure therapist.
- You must consult a doctor before using these points if you have any complications in your pregnancy.

SP6 You will find this point at the back of your shinbone above the ankle bone around 4 centimeters (1½ inches) upwards on the inside of your leg. Apply firm pressure with your index finger on the point for a few seconds. Take a break of one minute and then repeat. This point is excellent for speeding up labor and also for relieving pain.	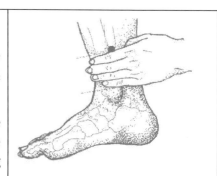
LI4 You will find this point in the webbing of the index finger between the thumb and index finger. Applying gentle pressure to it with the thumb of your other hand, and massaging it for a few moments will help to induce labor and also relieve labor pain.	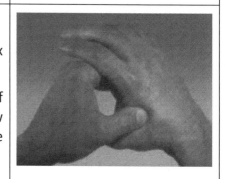

Massaging the hand from the elbow to the back side of the palm is also helpful in speeding up the labor process.

This needs to be a deep massage and can be given for 10-12 minutes.

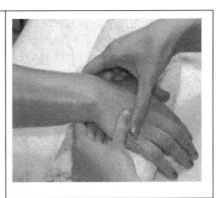

Points for reducing anxiety and pain during labor

K1

You can find this point in the center of the ball of your foot

This point helps to reduce anxiety, relaxes the body and calms the mind. It also helps the mother to maintain focus.

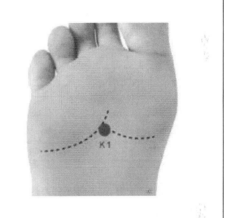

LI4

You will find this point in the webbing of the index finger between the thumb and index finger.

Applying gentle pressure to it with the thumb of your other hand, and massaging it for a few moments will help to induce labor and also relieve labor pain.

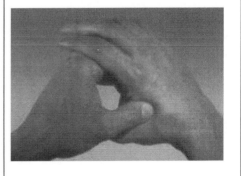

5.4 Points for the postnatal period

Acupressure can bring about a lot of positive changes to your health after the baby birth. Some of the most common postnatal issues that can be resolved with acupressure treatment are as follows:

Points for Postnatal Depression

One of the greatest difficulties that new mothers face is postpartum depression and anxiety. Using acupressure is the best natural way to come out of it, rather than depending on antidepressant medications. Stimulating the following points can help relieve this issue.

Use all the points shown in the 'Hormonal Imbalance' section above, plus the following ones.

HT7 You can find this point at the end of the wrist crease, on a line directly below the little finger. Stimulate it by applying moderate pressure using your thumb for two to three minutes twice a day. It is renowned for postnatal recovery and calming the mind and the spirit and bringing about harmony in the emotions. It is also useful in treating insomnia, sleeping disorders, panic, nausea as well as emotional and psychological issues.	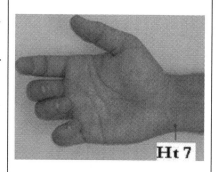
PC6 You can find this point at three finger's width above the wrist crease, right between the two tendons on the inner side of the forearm. Use moderate pressure for 2-3 minutes twice a day. This point opens the pathway to the heart and has a powerful calming and soothing effect on the spirit. It helps to alleviate stress and anxiety. It is also useful in treating asthma, vomiting, palpitations and poor memory.	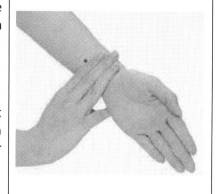

Point for Breast Tenderness

After delivery if the mother can't provide breastmilk for her baby for some reason then the breasts get engorged and cause pain. In such a situation following is the best point to stimulate.

You can locate this point just on the center on the back of your palm.

Press the point with your thumb for 4-5 minutes twice or thrice a day until you feel relief. Use a deep circular massage in this area.

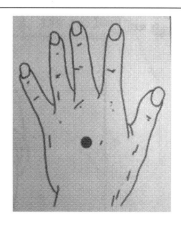

Point for Increasing Lactation

Sometimes the mother may suffer from insufficient milk production leading her to worry and feel stressful, but acupressure can help alleviate this problem in a natural and permanent way. At the same time, you should also use the remedies to increase lactation given in the chapter -8 'All about Breast and Breastfeeding'.

SI1

You will find this point at the corner of the nail on the outside of the little finger.

Press this point on both little fingers one after the other with a moderate pressure for 2-3 minutes, thrice a day. One can even use jimmy to press point.

Stimulating this point on both little fingers can help in treating insufficient lactation, breast abscess, mastitis and cysts.

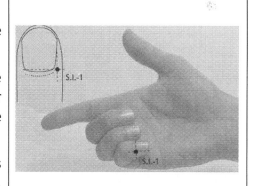

Point for Reducing Postnatal Belly

You can find this point four figures down from your belly button.

Press this point for up to 30-50 counts in circular motion twice a day.

This point reduces postnatal belly, improves digestion and corrects intestinal movement.

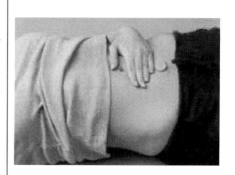

Points for Reducing Postnatal Fat

You will probably be carrying more fat than you used to after the baby is born. To reduce this postnatal fat, stimulating each point for 2-3 minutes twice a day with each hand.

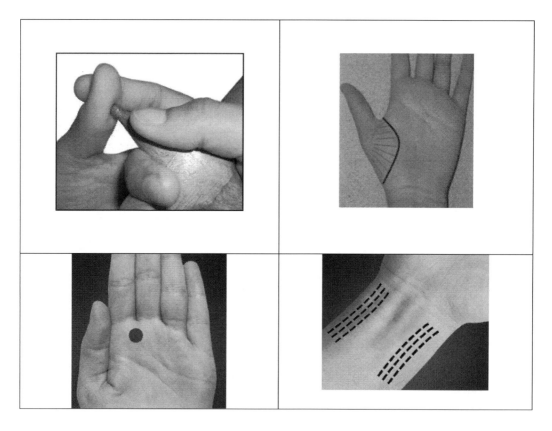

5.5 Points to Use for Baby

Here are some excellent points which you can use on your baby safely. Remember to use a very gentle pressure on them in a massaging movement, just as if you were playing with the baby.

To Ease Colic

Using your thumb, lightly press the esophagus reflex area, located in the ball of the foot, to ease colic pain.

Massage the area lightly for 30-40 seconds and then do the same on the other foot. You should also use the remedies indicated in Chapter 10 for colic pain.

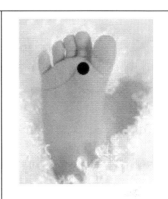

For Diarrhea

Gently press your thumb on the colon reflex area to treat diarrhea, and gently massage this area for 30-40 seconds once a day on one of the baby's feet, and repeat this on the baby's other foot. But if the condition is worse, massage both feet twice a day. You must consult a doctor if the baby has heavy diarrhea.

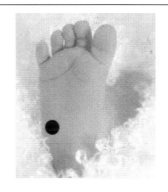

To Calm the Baby

To calm your baby, gently press your thumb on the solar plexus reflex area in the webbing of one of the baby's hands for 30-40 seconds, and repeat it on the other hand.

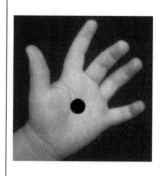

•••

This concludes the chapter on acupressure points you can use throughout your pregnancy, labor and beyond for treating various problems associated with these times. Now, let's move to labor in detail when the dear baby is born.

All about Labor and the early hours afterwards

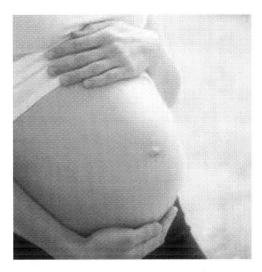

Generally, women think that giving birth to a child is a very painful and difficult process. But this is not right. I'm not saying that it is totally painless. Yes, you will feel pain but it will be bearable, and at the end you get to meet your baby, certainly the most beautiful gift in the world.

I really believe that every mother-to-be must have full knowledge of the labor process, and what she is expected to do at various stages in it to make it easier and better for both herself and her baby. Though it is a natural process, and a mother-to-be can give birth to a child even without proper knowledge, it is always better to have apt knowledge which will benefit not only herself but also her baby.

Benefits of having apt knowledge

When you know what is going to happen in labor, and what you are expected to do at what time, you can make sure that you are prepared beforehand and ready for what will happen.

Sometimes it is believed that a prepared state of mind will make you worry more, raise your stress levels and make you anxious or fearful during labor. But that is not true. A prepared state of mind...

- leads to a lack of tension in your muscles
- which leads to relaxed and loose muscles
- which leads to an appropriate oxygen supply in the muscles along with proper blood circulation
- which means the muscles work better
- which leads to less pain and an easy delivery!

This is an altogether better position to be in!

Handicaps of not having apt knowledge

When contractions start and you feel pain, an unprepared mind...
- leads to stress, anxiety or fear because of your lack of proper knowledge
- which leads to tightness in your muscles
- which leads to less oxygen in your muscles and poor blood flow
- which makes it difficult for your muscles to work
- which leads to even more pain and delays labor

And this is not the position you want to be in!

To help you understand the whole labor process, in this chapter we will discuss some very important topics like signs of labor, three stages of labor, some excellent remedies when complications occur, care of mother and the baby just after delivery and many more things.

6.1   Signs of Labor

The labor process is divided into three stages, each of which can be identified and understood by its own peculiar symptoms, or by a physical examination done by your doctor.

Early Signs of the Commencement of Labor

Usually when we think about labor, we are thinking about the final (relatively short) stage during which the baby is actually born. However, birth is the culmination of a long and complex process that begins much before the final birthing stage.

Labor usually begins before the mother-to-be is even aware that it has begun, but the following are few early indicators that it will begin, and they may appear up to 2-8 days before the actual labor.

- The mother-to-be feels ease in breathing compared to before.
- The upper part of her abdomen becomes a little soft as the fetus moves down towards the pelvis and the shape of her abdomen changes.
- She feels a lightness and freshness in her body.
- She feels the baby moving down.
- She feels emptiness on both lateral sides of her abdomen.
- She may have an urge to urinate or defecate frequently, because the baby is moving down.

[**Note**: If you are suffering from chronic constipation you will be highly susceptible to frequent defecation. It's always advisable to keep a check on constipation and if necessary use remedies for it.]

Signs that labor is just about to start

You should observe some other signs that will let you know that labor is about to start. According to the Ayurvedic text, *Astangraday Sharirsthan*, the mother-to-be might notice:

- Heaviness in lower parts
- Frequent urination
- Pain in back, abdomen, waist, pelvis, heart, thigh joints and vagina
- Watery or sticky discharge from vagina

And then contractions start.

Not all women experience all the above symptoms - some may experience only a few. Others may experience just a slight pain in their back before their water breaks and contractions start. It is different from woman to woman.

False labor pain

Lower abdominal pain can be considered as the major sign of the commencement of labor, but it may not necessarily be labor pain.

Sometimes a woman might be tricked into thinking that labor is about to start, when in fact the indicative pain is only indigestion or gas. This is called false labor pain and leads to unnecessary havoc, so it is important to know the difference between true and false labor pains.

True Labor Pains	False Labor Pains
The pain starts in the lower abdomen and slowly spreads to the genitals.	Pain occurs only in the abdomen above the naval.
The intensity of the pain gradually increases.	The intensity of the pain does not increase.
There is a watery discharge from the vagina, which is sometimes sticky or reddish colored.	There is no vaginal discharge.

You might recall from chapter-1 that the cervix remains closed through the pregnancy, but of course, it has to open up during labor so the fetus can first pass through it, then through the vagina and at last emerge from the external vaginal opening. These three separate things cover the three stages of labor.

Signs that it is time to go to hospital

You may have mild, irregular contractions for days before labor starts, but do not rush to the hospital unless you have an obvious complication, such as the baby is in breech position or you have been booked for a cesarean section (C-section). Just enjoy the excitement of knowing that things are probably starting to happen, but at the same time remain at peace yourself. Keep walking as much as possible, at the same time be gentle with yourself and conserve your energy by eating, drinking and resting in the comfort of your home.

Keeping calm is the key to coping with labor. There is no need to worry, as you are well prepared and your body knows what to do. The longer you stay at home the better, even though it is natural to be excited about going to the hospital. But being there does not mean that your baby will arrive any quicker, and in fact, many women find that their contractions stop once they get there, because anxiety inhibits contractions.

Once your contractions are strong and the gap between two contractions is about 10 minutes, or your water breaks, then it's the right time to go to the hospital. But remain relaxed, as there is still a lot of time for the delivery. Before going to the hospital though, you need to massage yourself with *Til* (sesame) oil to aid lubrication of your muscles, as that is good for their further expansion. It also strengthens your body and helps it relax. After that you should take a bath with warm water, and after dressing you should consume some specially prepared herbal tea (the liquid food preparation that follows).

Preparation of herbal tea

This tea increases your body's strength and encourages proper contractions. Mix the following powdered herbs in equal quantity: *asheriyo* (common cress) + *suthi* (dry ginger) + *taj* (cinnamon) + *akkalgaro* (Anacyclus pyrethrum dc.) + *tejbal* (toothache tree).

Put a pan on the stove and add 25 gm of ghee. Mix 10 gm of the above powdered mixture and sauté it for 30 seconds on low flame. Add 25 gm of jaggery + 1 glass of water. Boil it well and your tea is ready. Have it hot.

We'll discuss the three stages of labor in detail now, understand different things that will be happening in each of them, and what you will be doing in each one.

6.2 Three Stages of Labor

First Stage: Effacement and Dilation

In the first stage the elastic tissues of your uterus start to become thin ('efface') and your cervix opens (dilates). A totally dilated cervix marks the end of this first stage.

In this stage, contractions start very mild and gradually increase in intensity. Contractions happen because the uterus starts tightening and shortening in its upper portion and as a result, the baby starts to move downwards towards the cervix.

In this stage you will notice a sticky or bloody discharge from your vagina.

Once the contractions become regular with intervals of 10 minutes between them, you can go to the hospital.

There are three phases of Stage 1.

(1A) During the first phase of Stage 1, the contractions become more regular and slightly more intense (but still easily within your toleration), as the cervix starts to dilate (open). These contractions may last for 30-60 seconds with irregular intervals of 5-20 minutes between them. It is best if you are walking around or doing normal household work during this phase.

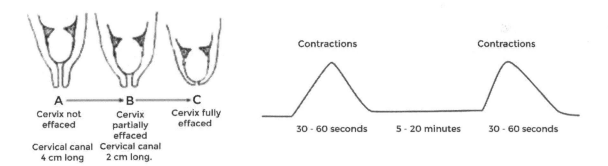

A — Cervix not effaced — Cervical canal 4 cm long
B — Cervix partially effaced — Cervical canal 2 cm long.
C — Cervix fully effaced

Contractions — 30 - 60 seconds — 5 - 20 minutes — 30 - 60 seconds — Contractions

(1B) In the second phase of Stage 1, the contractions last for 1 minute with intervals of 5 minutes between them, your cervix opens up to 7 cm and there is a watery discharge from your vagina. This phase lasts 5 to 9 hours in the first pregnancy, and 2-5 hours in subsequent pregnancies. During this phase, you can walk around if you like, but if that's inconvenient because of pain you can adopt one of the yoga postures given at the end of Chapter 3, as they are likely to be less painful – it's really up to you to choose what suits you best.

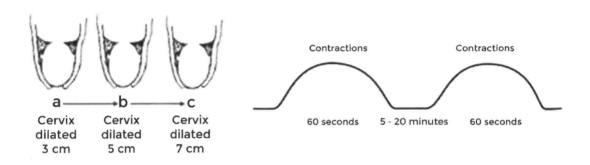

a————▸b————▸c		
Cervix dilated 3 cm	Cervix dilated 5 cm	Cervix dilated 7 cm

Contractions   Contractions

60 seconds   5 - 20 minutes   60 seconds

(1C) In the third phase of Stage 1, the contractions continue to become more intense and you may struggle to control yourself, but breathing exercises will help you the best. Here your water may break though it's more likely that it'll rupture some time during active labor (i.e. in the second stage of labor). Your cervix will open to its full capacity of 7-10 cm, and the contractions last for 1-1.5 minutes with intervals of 3-4 minute between them. The good news is that the total duration of this phase is very short.

During this phase, you might not be able to walk, so if that is the case this is the best time to use the yoga postures given in Chapter 3, Section 3.5, to ease the pain and also to get the advantage of gravity to encourage the baby into the right position.

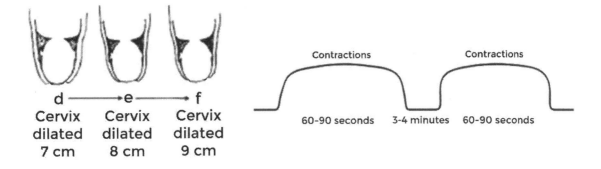

d ———→e———→ f

| Cervix dilated 7 cm | Cervix dilated 8 cm | Cervix dilated 9 cm |

A fully dilated cervix marks the end of the first stage of labor.

Phase (1A) and (1B) are easily bearable, but Phase (1C) requires more strength.

The total duration of Stage 1 is generally 12-24 hours, but you should be aware that some women don't feel Phases (1A) and (1B) and directly feel Phase (1C), so for them the total duration of Stage 1 is very short.

Note:
- During Stage 1 you may have the urge to push the fetus out, before the cervix is fully dilated. Do not give in to this urge since the baby's head may press on the un-dilated cervix and cause swelling in the cervical area.
- Always ask your doctor if it is okay for you to start pushing! You will be given the 'all clear' when your cervix is fully dilated.

Second Stage: Delivery

Stage 2 starts when your cervix is full dilated and ends with the birth of your baby.

During Stage 1 of labor, it is advisable for you to be mobile, but in Stage 2 you will be moved to the labor room and advised to lie down. The rupture of the amniotic sac occurs at this time, but as the head of the fetus blocks the birth canal, not all of the amniotic fluid is expelled. The remaining fluid helps to create pressure and helps the baby to move down the birth canal (vagina).

Stage 2 is the time when you can actively participate in the labor process. Whenever you feel a contraction, push downwards and continue to push until the contraction stops. This will add to the effectiveness of the contractions in pushing the baby down the birth canal, and also in easing your pain. Pushing before or after a contraction is ineffective and makes you tired.

According to one of the oldest known Ayurveda texts, *Charaka Samhita*, contractions generally occur at intervals of 2-3 minutes and last for 1-1.5 minutes. Breathe deeply and calm yourself as much as possible during the interval between contractions, so that you are peaceful and relaxed before the next contraction.

In general, Stage 2 lasts about 30 minutes to 1 hour.

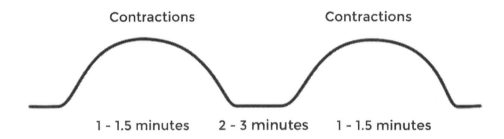

Contractions   Contractions

1 - 1.5 minutes   2 - 3 minutes   1 - 1.5 minutes

Third Stage: Removing the Placenta

Once the baby is born, the uterus rests for 15-20 minutes and then contractions starts again, this time to expel the placenta, which is attached to the uterine wall. This time contractions will have low intensity, and you are not required to push. The placenta should not be pulled out as that may cause injury.

The placenta is a very important organ. It enables the fetus to breathe, receive nutrition from its mother's body, and grow from an embryo to a fully developed fetus, ready to be born. Its length equals the length of the baby which can be up to 46-61 cm (18-24 inches).

The expulsion of the placenta is a natural process, which happens within 30 minutes or so after the baby's birth. In case the placenta does not come out then, the following section contains a few Ayurvedic remedies to help.

6.3   Difficulties and remedies during labor

We'll deal with two types of labor and their related difficulties.

- Normal labor and its difficulties
- Abnormal labor

Normal Labor and its Difficulties

In this kind of labor all the factors for normal delivery are present – the baby's position is correct, and the mother's pelvis, cervix or vagina are properly developed. Sometimes though, there might be a few difficulties which can constrict easy natural labor.

- Weak contractions
- Delayed expulsion of the placenta.

Weak Contractions

Sometimes the mother has only light contractions which do not increase in strength over time and continue like this for 12-13 hours, or even longer. At other times, the contractions increase in strength, but suddenly decrease even though the cervix is not fully dilated. In both cases, labor is delayed and the mother suffers.

Strong contractions are required for a successful normal delivery, and thankfully, Ayurveda has some remedies to aid or restart good contractions naturally.

- Chew *tamalpatra* (bay leaf) or smoke the vagina with *tamalpatra* (bay leaf).
- Take a hip bath in water in which the herb *heela bol* (myrrh) is dissolved.
- Grind *pipli* (Indian long pepper) + *vaja* (*Acorus calamus*) in water and prepare a paste. Add this paste to castor oil and apply this smooth paste to your navel.
- Smoke the vagina with *hing* (asafetida).
- According to the naturopath, Louise Kunhe, a hip bath works excellently in this situation. If you can't take one, you can put a mud pack below your navel and change it after every 1-2 hours. And if this is also not possible, you can use a very cold compression on your navel and also on your breast.

Delayed Expulsion of the Placenta

If the placenta is not naturally expelled on its own, Ayurveda has some helpful remedies.

- Mix equal volumes of *til* (sesame) oil + Turpentine and use it to massage the navel and below with a downward movement.
- Smoke the mother's vaginal area using *bhojpatra* (Himalayan birch) and *guggal* (*Commiphora mukul*)
- Apply a paste made from the finely ground root of the *kalalavi* (Gloriosa Superba) to the woman's palm and soles.

Abnormal labor

Abnormal labor happens when the mother-to-be has some physical defects, or the fetus is in an inappropriate position in the uterus.

The physical defects might be that the reproductive organs of the mother-to-be are not properly developed, or her vagina or pelvic girdle are narrow, or her cervix is inappropriately shaped. The fetus will be in an inappropriate position if it is in breech position, or if its legs, rather than its head, is downwards, or if it is in some other position in which normal delivery is not possible.

In all the above cases a caesarean section is required. You can see some pictures in the next chapter to get a clear idea about this topic.

6.4   Cutting the Cord

Let's go back a bit at the end of Stage 2, when the baby is just born. It is still connected to the umbilical cord from its umbilicus (naval), the other end of which is connected to the mother's uterine wall. Now, it's time to cut the cord.

Ayurveda has sound advice about how to do this. According to its ancient text, *Sushruta Samhita*, the mucus covering the newborn's face, eyes, mouth and nose should be removed first, because this hinders the working of its respiratory system, at the very time when the baby is trying to take its first breath after birth.

Crying signals the commencement of its respiration, and if this occurs immediately that is an indication of the baby's good health. But if the baby does not cry, here are some safe practices that can be used to make it cry.

- Pour reasonably cold and hot water alternatively on the baby. Be careful while doing this.
- Gently pat the baby's back, thigh or cheek.

- Initiate artificial respiration if necessary.

Once the baby is breathing satisfactorily, it is time to cut the cord.

To prepare for this, according to *Charaka Samhita*, once the baby has started crying properly, a small cotton swab dipped in pure ghee should be placed, or wiped very gently, on the fontanel (crown chakra).

To cut the cord, the *Charaka Samhita* continues, tightly tie a piece of silk thread at a distance of 8 fingers (about 4-5 inches/10-12 cm) from the baby's umbilicus, and then a second piece a little distance away from the first thread. Then check the pulse on the cord between the two threads, and when it has stopped pulsating, it is the right time to cut the umbilical cord with a sterile sharp instrument.

If the baby is weak, you can lower its upper body slightly to let all the blood drain from the placenta into its body. You can even rub the cord downwards towards the baby to move the blood from the cord into the baby, and then the cord can be safely cut.

After a few days the cord remaining attached to the baby's umbilicus will dry out and drop off. If it gets swollen, please check *Remedies for Common Problems* in Chapter 10, *Baby Care*.

6.5 Care of the Baby after Delivery

After birth, the baby needs some immediate care, just like the mother after labor. Actually both these treatments occur simultaneously. But for now, let's first look at the baby's early care.

After the baby has started breathing and after its cord has been cut, it's time to give the baby a bath to clean off all the fat and mucus deposited on it.

In preparation for the bath, it is recommended to gently apply a specially prepared oil (see below) all over the baby's skin, to facilitate the easy removal of the sticky mucus substances in the bath. The oil also checks water from penetrating baby's skin, thus preventing it from getting cold, and helps to maintain the baby's body temperature.

For the bath, it is always good to use lukewarm water. Using *besan* (chickpea flour), rather than soap is a good idea too.

Oil preparation

Take 100 gm of coconut oil + 10 gm of *nirgundi* (*Vitex nigundo*) leaves + 5 gm *ajwain* (carom seeds). Boil, strain and use the oil obtained.

Water preparation

- If affordable, the water used to bathe the baby can be prepared as follows:
  Put 5-10 gm of gold biscuit + 10-15 gm of silver biscuit in the bathing water and boil it for a few minutes.
  Remove the gold and silver biscuits and let the water cool down till it is lukewarm and suitable for bathing the baby. Such a bath is thought to increase the lifespan of the baby.

- According to Ayurveda there is another suitable preparation for bathing water which pacifies *vata*.
  Boil the bath water with following herbs:
  taj (cinnamon) + bay leaves + cardamom + *lavang* (clove) + *kapoor* (camphor) + *Nagkeshar* bark or leaves (Mesua ferrea) + *Kankol* (allspice) + *shilajeet* (a thick, sticky tar like substance found in the Himalayan & Tibetan mountains). Let the water cool down till it is lukewarm and suitable to bathe the baby in.

Alternatively, make a decoction (mash and then boil) of the above herbs and add them to the lukewarm bathing water.

After the bath the baby is ready and may be hungry, so it's time for *Gadthuthi/Jatkarma Sanskar* (baby's first feed) which is the topic of the last section.

If you feel that the baby is hungry just after birth, you can feed it with *Gadthuthi* before the oiling and bathing.

6.6   Care of the mother just after delivery

After the third stage of labor, the new mother is very weak, sensitive and exhausted. Gently clean her genitals with warm water, and then tie an abdominal belt around her abdomen. This helps the uterus to return to its original shape. It also prevents backache, flatulence and a loose abdomen.

The next thing is to cover her ears with a scarf, and possibly place small balls of cotton in her ears to prevent them getting exposed to wind or cold air from a fan or air conditioner.

Now it is time for her to rest. After a lot of exhausting labor, she really requires a deep and sound sleep without any interruption. By taking 4-6 hour of sleep now, preferably on the back, she re-charges.

Congratulations! You've done a great job to get to this point and you've got the most beautiful gift in the world. Enjoy this feeling to the fullest. Drink in your baby with your eyes till you are satisfied. Hold your baby in your hands and heart, and speak lovingly to it. You are the only person it knows and recognizes, so it is you that it needs!

After you arise, you may feel hungry, but you should pass urine before you eat. Urination should occur within 5-8 hour of the labor finishing, but if it does not, then place a hot water-bottle or a heated heat-pack on your abdomen. If urination still does not occur, you must consult a doctor. Once your urinary system is functioning again properly, you can eat. Here are some good recipes for this first meal.

1. Mix 2.5 gm *suthi* (dry ginger powder) + 10 gm ghee + 10 gm jaggery together and consume first.
2. Consume some *Raab* (check recipe section in chapter 12 - Miscellaneous)

In all of this, you need to be very careful with your body and avoid even a single jerk. You will not be able to sit for a long time, and are advised to lie down on your back for at least 3 days.

6.7 Gadthuthi (Baby's first feed)

Gadthuthi is an ancient word, which is also known as *jatakarma sanskar*, and it refers to the baby's first feed. It is composed of two words, *gad* (sweetness) and *thuthi* (bitter taste), because *gadthuthi* is a preparation combining these two.

At this point, the question needs to be explored about why something other than breast milk might be given to the baby for its first feed. There are a number of reasons, but still, there is no strict rule, so it's your choice about whether to give your baby Gadthuthi or breast milk for its first feed.

- Because you have just passed through the process of labor, a lot of stress hormones are floating around in your blood and body, so according to Ayurveda it's not the right time to feed your baby as your blood directly affects the quality of your breast milk. It is always better for you to have a proper sleep of 4-6 hours just after delivery to allow your stress levels to reduce and to allow you to re-charge. During that time, Gadthuthi works well.

- If you are still in the labor room for stitches or cleaning, and the baby is hungry Gadthuthi facilitates the situation.
- If you have a C-section, a lot of time is spent in the operating theater after the baby is delivered, so during that time Gadthuthi is also a helpful source for a first feed.
- Gadthuthi also has benefits in its own right, which are listed in the two recipes below.

According to Ayurveda this *sanskar* (tradition) is one of the most important ones, and should be performed as soon as possible. You can use any of the following three recipes:

Gadthuthi Recipe 1

In earlier times, *Gadthuthi* was made of three things, a piece of *gud* (jaggery) about the size of a chickpea + 3-4 drops of ghee + 1 *neem* leaf. Mix these with 1 cup of water, boil and strain. The resulting water is called Gadthuthi, and it can be given to the baby with the help of small a spoon. There are scientific benefits of this too, thus making it an excellent first food for the new born babies.

- *Gud* strengthens the heart of the fetus, cleans the blood, helps the kidneys, and also works as a very mild laxative.
- *Neem* expels excess heat from the body, helps its intestines, and also works as a very good anti–infection agent.
- Ghee smooths the intestines and softly removes old stools.

Gadthuthi Recipe 2

This recipe is described in the *Sushruta Samhita,* an ancient Ayurvedic text.

Put one drop of pure honey + two drops of ghee on a grindstone (marble / granite stone specially prepared for grinding herbs). Take a piece of pure gold (i.e. 24 carat) biscuit (even 1 gm is sufficient), but not jewelry, and grind it in a clockwise circle on the mixture. Then gently rub this mixture on to the baby's tongue, with the ring finger of your right hand. Note that the quantities of ghee and honey should never be the same as that is poisonous.

- Honey works wonder on the baby's lungs, and it also improves its immune system.
- Ghee lubricates the body and intestines, and makes its stool easy to excrete.
- Gold increases the baby's lifespan, intellect and memory.

Gadthuthi Recipe 3

If you can't obtain a gold biscuit you can use just honey and water, where you mix together twice as much water as honey (such as 1 teaspoon honey + 2 teaspoons water) and give to the baby on a small spoon.

....

So here we conclude the chapter on labor and the hours following it.

In it you have found out what happens during the labor process that will wonderfully result in you meeting your baby in person. Having knowledge of the three stages of the process will enable you to accept each stage with something closer to equanimity, rather than fear of the unknown, and this of course will minimize any stress that both you and your baby may experience. It is after all a natural process, and your being able to go with the flow as much as possible will be better for both of you.

You've also found out what should be done in the hours following your baby's birth to provide the best care possible for the one who has just been pushed out of its watery haven into the birth canal and then out into this world, and for the one whose body made such a mammoth effort by doing all that pushing. We turn next to what modern science says about pregnancy and labor, so that you can find out about the modern practices that will be applied to you, as well as those you might require for some complication – but hopefully won't.

What Modern Science Says

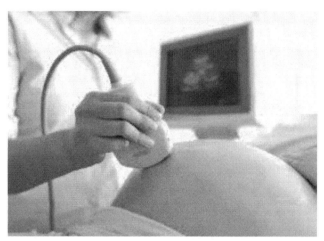

This chapter provides information about pregnancy and labor from the perspective of modern science. For instance, once it is confirmed that you are pregnant, the hospital's process will be set in motion, which initially means that they will ask you to have a few tests done. Using information from here you will be able to visualize what will happen in the labor room if you have a normal labor or an assisted delivery. In which condition c-section is required and what happens in a c-section in case you need it. Terms such as episiotomy and epidural and so on are described so you know what they mean.

7.1 Investigations during Pregnancy

Nowadays, being pregnant will involve you in quite a few tests, (beginning from confirming the pregnancy to checking the final position and health of the baby right before the delivery) not only to find out right at the start whether you are really pregnant or not, but also to check your and your baby's health throughout pregnancy. As you go through the motions of various tests, talk to your doctor and figure out the most necessary ones and try to opt out of others. The lesser the pricking and prodding, the better your anxiety levels. Have as few tests as possible, only the necessary ones.

Pregnancy Tests
Pregnancy test kits are readily available in supermarkets or at chemists. You can easily use one of these, and resolve your curiosity in the comfort of your home, and hopefully get the result if you wish. Nowadays, they are more than 99% accurate if used correctly.

Blood Tests
When your pregnancy is confirmed, having your blood tested is one of the first routine tests in order to check various things like...

Blood Group

It is vital to know your blood group in case of an emergency, and also for your Rh factor. If you have Rh negative blood, and your partner has Rh positive blood (or vice versa), the baby's blood can be either positive or negative. If you have a positive blood group and your baby has a negative blood group, no risk is posed while you are pregnant. However, if you have a negative blood group and your baby has a positive one, there may be a risk which requires a necessary but precautionary treatment.

Hemoglobin Level

While you are pregnant you are susceptible to low hemoglobin levels (the molecule in red blood cells that carries oxygen) since you are nourishing both yourself and the baby, so if there are signs of anemia, because the hemoglobin level is low, it must be corrected. The required level of hemoglobin should be 11-12 g/dl.

Blood Sugar

There may be some fluctuation in your blood sugar levels due to changes in carbohydrate metabolism. It is very important that your sugar level is monitored on a regular basis, if there is an existing family history of diabetes, or even sudden weight gain. A high blood sugar level does not always mean that you have diabetes, but it is always better to control your sugar level by correcting your diet and by using acupressure. (Please refer to Chapter 5.)

HIV and Hepatitis B

Hepatitis B is a liver disease that can be easily passed to your baby, you can transmit it to your infant during childbirth. If you are positive for Hepatitis B, then your baby will require two shots soon after birth which will easily prevent it from acquiring this infection.

Repeated use of the same syringe, or by blood transfusion of infected blood, or unprotected extra marital sex leads to AIDS infection. Even if your test is positive, with proper treatment, if it is detected early enough, the fetus can be protected from being HIV infected.

Rubella

It is advisable to have a Rubella vaccination before you conceive (and then wait for at least 3 months before you start trying to conceive). If you are pregnant and have not been immunized against Rubella, this shot can't be given during pregnancy, but your doctor will give it to you after your delivery. This is important because if you get infected with Rubella, it can get transmitted to your fetus.

Blood Pressure

If you have high blood pressure, it can affect the growth of your baby, and also develop into a life threatening condition for both of you. So your blood pressure should be checked at every visit, especially in the last trimester.

Urine

You will be advised to have your urine checked for two things.

Sugar

If sugar is found in your urine, you will have to change your diet.

Albumin (blood serum)

If your albumin level is abnormally high, it can affect the nutritional status of the fetus. High levels of albumin can also be a sign of pre-eclampsia, if it is accompanied by a rise in blood pressure, or swelling around the eyes, burning or a frequent urge to urinate and a white discharge. Please seek doctor's advice if its level is high, as pre-eclampsia can be very dangerous for both you and the fetus.

Ultrasound Scans/Sonography

When you go for a scan, the person doing the scan will initially rub a special gel onto your abdomen to reduce signal loss from the probe. Then the probe will be placed on your abdomen and slid around on the gel. The reflected ultrasound waves create a picture on a screen, which shows solid structures as white and liquid structures as black.

This test tells you many things about the condition of the fetus, such as whether it has any deformities or genetic defects, the position of the umbilical cord, whether you are having twins or a single child, and also the dimensions and measurements of the child's head, arm, hands and other external physical organs.

These days, ultrasound scans have become the norm and doctors generally perform it at almost every appointment. In general, this is not required. The initial scan to determine your pregnancy and the 3D scans at 20 weeks and 36 weeks are necessary but try and avoid the ultrasounds to be monthly happening. Talk to your doctor to chart out a satisfactory plan for both them and you regarding the scans. Of course, due to complications it might become inevitable for the doctor to perform regular scans, but unnecessary repetitions for any other reason, like checking the growth of the baby, should be avoided.

7.2 Assisted Deliveries

Forceps and ventouse (vacuum extraction) are two types of assisted deliveries, in which instruments are used to assist with the birth of your baby. They can only be used during Stage 2 of labor. If your baby needs to be born quickly before Stage 2, it will be delivered by an emergency caesarean birth. An obstetrician performs both these types of delivery.

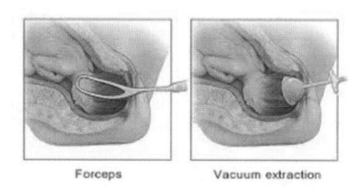

Forceps   Vacuum extraction

Reasons for Assisted delivery

An assisted delivery is commonly done if you have been pushing for a long time and your baby is making slow (or little) progress down the birth canal, and particularly if the baby is showing signs of distress. Slow progress during stage 2 is more likely if it was already slow during stage 1, perhaps indicating that you have a large baby or that the baby's head is not in the right position.

Ventouse

A ventouse uses suction to help guide your baby out. A metal or plastic cup is attached to your baby's head by suction, which comes from a machine via a tube. You push with each contraction as usual, and the obstetrician gently pulls the cup, thus helping your baby out. It is not always necessary to have an episiotomy with this procedure.

Forceps

Forceps are a pair of metal instruments that look rather like two large linked salad servers and are placed inside the vagina. They cradle the baby's head and guide it out, although you still need to push with the contractions. With a forceps delivery, the mother usually has a local anesthetic or an epidural.

Forceps, also known as Kielland Forceps, are used to help turn your baby, if it is facing the wrong way. An episiotomy is not always necessary for this, but is performed in many cases to help the baby's delivery.

Effects of an assisted delivery on your baby

An assisted delivery can cause distress or trauma to your baby, so a pediatrician is usually there in the labor room too. Babies who've had a ventouse delivery commonly have a bump on the back of their head that is usually reddish purple in color and can be quite prominent. Forceps can sometimes leave two red marks on the sides of your baby's head, but any bruises or bumps normally go down within the first week. Because of the bruising, these babies are more likely to develop jaundice. If a baby appears irritable after an instrumental delivery, it may be best not to let too many different people handle it for the time being.

7.3 Episiotomy

An episiotomy is a small cut made at the entrance of your vagina (on your perineum) to give your baby more room during the birth. According to Ayurveda, an episiotomy is not always necessary, but it is more likely to be needed for an instrumental delivery. Nowadays, the main reason for an episiotomy is the need for quick delivery and it is carried out routinely without really assessing if it is needed or not. Normally, the mouth of the vagina is optimally dilated and relaxed at this stage, so the baby can come out easily.

An episiotomy is not very painful as the area is very thin at the height of a contraction, and the incision is made with one quick snip of a pair of sterile scissors. Due to this the mother may also have a few stitches.

7.4 Epidural

An epidural is a medication which brings relief to pain from the waist down by numbing the area. A fine tube is inserted by an anesthetist into the base of the spine, through which an anesthetic is introduced, which can either be topped up as required, or given continuously by an infusion pump. According to Ayurveda, epidurals should not be used as they numb the lower area and the mother is not able to feel contractions and is therefore not able to push at the right time. They also slow down contractions which are highly inappropriate.

Advantages
An epidural can lower the mother's blood pressure if it is very high (a good thing), but this drop will not affect the baby unless her blood pressure drops below the normal range. It is also good in cases where the mother is suffering from intense pain and exhausted from extremely long labor and the labor is not progressing.

Disadvantages
An anesthetist needs to be available to administer an epidural. The mother must keep still while it is administered, which is very difficult during a contraction. The mother may need to be catheterized, which means that a drip is set up in case her blood pressure falls. There is the risk of severe headache. If the needle accidentally pierces the sheath around the spinal cord, movement is severely or totally restricted.

7.5 When is a Caesarean Birth required?

There are two main reasons for having a planned caesarean birth (c section) – a medical condition or structural reason of the mother and the position of the baby in the uterus.

Medical conditions or structural reasons of the mother
A planned caesarean section will be required if the mother already suffers from a medical condition such as a heart problem, high blood pressure, diabetes, severe pre-eclampsia and the like, or if she has a structural problem like an inappropriate pelvic structure (see pic 1) or *placenta previa* (see pic 2) (the placenta is attached to the uterine wall very low near to the cervix), etc.

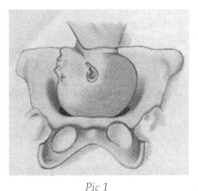

Pic 1

The pelvis is narrow, or the pelvis is normal but the baby's head is too large

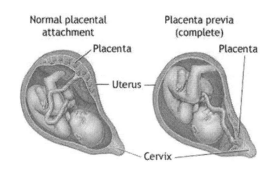

Pic 2

Position of baby in the uterus

The position of your baby in the uterus can affect the labor and birth. By the 36th week of pregnancy, most babies will have positioned their head down ready for labor - an ideal position for normal delivery. However, some babies move around and frequently change their position which is technically known as an "unstable lie".

Occiput anterior (OA)

This is the best position of a baby for normal and easy labor and majority of the babies adopt it. In this your baby will probably be facing your back, with its back slightly to one side of your abdomen. In medical terms this is called *occiput anterior* (occiput is the back of the baby's head) position. If the baby's back is on your right side, it's in the *right occiput anterior* (ROA) position, and if it is on your left, it's in the *left occiput anterior* (LOA) position.

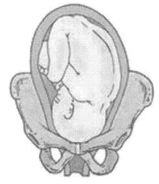

Left occiput anterior (LOA)

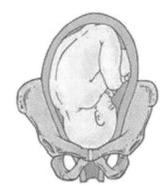

Right occiput anterior (ROA)

Occiput posterior (OP)

If the baby is facing your front with its back against your back, this is called an *occiput posterior* position. However, during labor they naturally take one of the OA positions. Only about 5 percent of these babies fail to move into OA. Their vaginal birth is also possible, but you may have a little more backache or a long labor and there are chances that you'll need an assisted delivery.

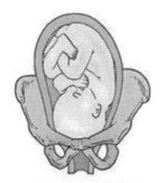

Left occiput posterior (LOP)

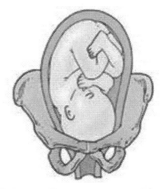

Right occiput posterior (ROP)

Breech

A breech position occurs when your baby's buttocks are facing down and its head is under your ribs (complete breech), its legs may be tucked up (a frank breech), one or both legs might be pointing down (a footling breech). For all of these, the obstetrician may try to manipulate your abdomen to try to turn the baby around, but if this does not work, you will require a caesarean.

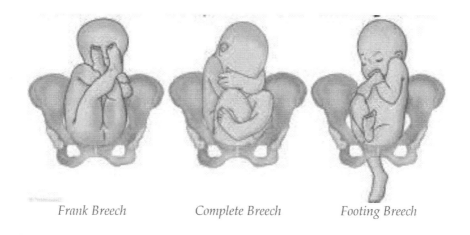

Frank Breech   *Complete Breech*   *Footing Breech*

Transverse lie

If your baby's head lies towards your left or right side, it means your baby is lying horizontally in your uterus (a transverse lie). Unless the baby turns, you will need a caesarean.

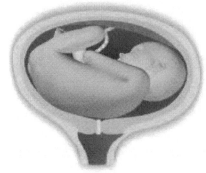

Transverse Lie

Reasons for needing an emergency or unplanned caesarean

Here are a few reasons for an emergency (unplanned) caesarean birth, but it still differs from doctor to doctor.

- Your baby becomes distressed during labor.
- Placenta abruption (the placenta comes adrift during labor) occurs.
- Labor does not progress, which means if it is very slow and very drawn out.
- The use of instruments such as forceps or ventouse is unsuccessful.
- The umbilical cord slips through your cervix ahead of your baby (prolapse of the cord). This means there's a danger that the cord will be squashed as your baby descends the cervix, thus cutting off its oxygen supply.

7.6   Augmenting or inducing labour

Generally, when your labor isn't progressing very well because of few irregular contractions, or if the contractions are ineffective in dilating the cervix and moving the baby down the birth canal, your healthcare practitioner may try to help stimulate your contractions. This practice is called augmenting or inducing labor. In it the doctor uses drugs to open the cervix. Augmentation of labor is required in other situations too, such as a post dated pregnancy (pregnancy overdue by 7-10 days), rupture of the membranes before labor has started, infection in the amniotic sac, and other such conditions.

Keep in mind though, that if induced labor is required, you should first try the options given in the remedy section 'Weak Contractions' in chapter 6, and also the acupressure points given in chapter 5 for this. Both of these are very safe and effective.

Let us also discuss inducing labor according to modern science, to keep you well informed. However, take this treatment only if it is absolutely necessary.

How is it done?
Before augmenting your labor, your practitioner will carefully assess the pattern of your contractions and examine you to find out how much your cervix has effaced (thinned out) and dilated, as well as how far your baby has descended. She'll also pay close attention to your baby's heart rate in response to the contractions you are having to make sure your baby will be able to tolerate stronger contractions. Then, if she determines that it's appropriate to augment your labor, there are two methods available – oxytocin or amniotomy.

Oxytocin
You'll be given a drug called oxytocin, which is a synthetic form of the hormone that your body naturally produces during spontaneous labor. You'll receive it through an IV line (Intravenous drip).
Your practitioner will start with a small dose and gradually increase it until your uterus responds appropriately. How much you'll need depends on the quality of your contractions so far, how sensitive your uterus is to the drug, how much your cervix is already dilated, and how far along you are in your pregnancy. As a rule, you're aiming at three to five contractions every ten minutes.
The goal is to give you just enough oxytocin to bring on contractions that dilate your cervix in a timely way and help your baby descend, but not so much that your contractions become too frequent or abnormally long and strong, which could stress your baby.

Risk factors for oxytocin
The most common problem associated with oxytocin is over stimulation of the uterus. This happens if the dosage is high, and it may in turn cause various problems with the baby's heart rate. But because oxytocin wears off pretty quickly, your practitioner can solve that problem by lowering the dose, or temporarily stopping the infusion altogether.

Amniotomy

Your practitioner can also try to expedite your labor by rupturing the membranes (the bag of waters) that surround the baby, if your waters haven't already broken on their own. This practice is beneficial only when your cervix is in a favourable condition (i.e. thinned out and dilated). She does this by inserting a slim, plastic hooked instrument through your vagina and the dilated cervix to rupture your amniotic sac. This should cause no more discomfort than a regular vaginal exam.

Risk factors for amniotomy

On the other hand, keeping your amniotic sac intact until it breaks on its own offers greater protection against infection and protection of the umbilical cord from compression during contractions.

Prerequisites for inducing labor

Before inducing labor some conditions must be fulfilled for an optimal subsequent labor.

- The cervix has started thinning out.
- The baby's head has descended into the birth canal.
- The amniotic fluid around the baby is adequate.
- All the factors are favorable for a normal delivery.

7.7 Caesarean Birth (C-section)

What if you need a caesarean birth? A caesarean birth is not different from any other operation. Your pubic hair will be shaved and the midwife will insert a catheter into your bladder just prior to the operation. A needle will be put into your hand through which fluid will drip if your blood pressure falls. It takes about 10 minutes from the first incision in your belly until the delivery of your baby and about another 40 minutes for the stitches in the combined layers of muscle, fat and skin. The procedure will not hurt you, but you will be aware that something is happening inside you. You will usually be given a spinal block or epidural so that you can stay awake during the operation and hold your baby soon afterwards (in my experience, you do feel the final push by the doctor right before the baby arrives).

After the birth, you are required a good rest as you've just had major surgery. It is always a good idea to ask your doctor or midwife to advise you about the sitting, feeding and sleeping positions which will help you. The recovery time after a C-section is much longer than that after a normal delivery, so electing to have a caesarean without any necessary medical ground, is not advisable.

7.8 Some terminologies

Here are some terms that you might come across during pregnancy or in the labor room.

Contractions:
A contraction is what happens when the uterine muscle tightens and relaxes to help your baby move down, pass through the uterus and later out of the birth canal.

Crowning:
During delivery, your baby's head will begin to show through your vaginal opening with each contraction. When your baby's head remains visible without slipping back in, it is known as "crowning".

Fetal Distress:
Fetal distress typically occurs when the fetus has not been receiving enough oxygen. It may occur when the pregnancy lasts too long, or when there are complications of pregnancy or labor. Usually, doctors identify fetal distress based on an abnormal heart rate in the fetus.

Placental Abruption:
Placental abruption is a complication of pregnancy, during which the placental lining is separated from the mother's uterus prior to delivery. It is the most common pathological cause of bleeding in late pregnancy.

Meconium:
Meconium is a greenish black substance that is present in the bowels of a growing fetus. It is normally discharged shortly after birth in the baby's first few bowel movements. Occasionally, it is discharged during labor, which may suggest that the fetus is distressed.

Water Breaking:
During pregnancy, your baby is surrounded and cushioned by a fluid filled membranous sac called the amniotic sac. At the beginning or during labor, the membranes will rupture, which is known as water breaking.

....

So this now concludes the chapter on what modern science says about pregnancy and labor.

In it, you learnt about the investigative tests that will be performed during your pregnancy, and the various procedures that can be used for an assisted delivery if you need it.

We now move to the subject of breasts and breast feeding in the next chapter, so you know best how to feed your new baby.

All about breasts and breastfeeding

Once your precious baby is born, you need to be able to breastfeed it successfully so it is properly nourished over the coming months. Once you become comfortable with breastfeeding, you'll both enjoy the closeness of this special time together and be happy knowing that this is the very best way to nourish your baby.

In This chapter will discuss everything about breasts and breastfeeding – structure of breasts, what changes occur during pregnancy, how to get hold of a perfect latch and different positions for feeding, about feeding chart, what to do if you find yourself with less flow of breast milk and many more things.

8.1   Structure and functioning of breasts.

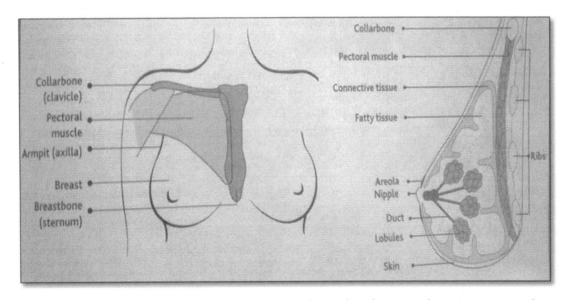

Each breast lies over the top of pectoral muscle in the chest, and its tissue extends downwards from below the collarbone down to the seventh rib, and outwards from the breastbone to the underarm. At the center of the breast is the nipple, surrounded by a brown pigmented region called the areola.

Breast tissue is composed of lobes, lobules and ducts, with each breast having about 15-20 lobes fanning out underneath the areola and nipple. These lobes are further divided into smaller lobules, which are linked by a system of ducts (tubes), which also lead directly to the nipple.

The main function of the breasts is to produce, store and release milk for feeding the baby. Milk is produced by the lobules when they are stimulated by hormones after childbirth, and is then carried by the ducts to the nipple, where it is passed to your baby for breastfeeding. Fat and connective tissue surrounds the ducts and lobules that shape the breasts. The areola both spread and darken a little during your pregnancy and contain small sweat glands which release a lubricant during breastfeeding.

8.2   Changes in breasts during pregnancy

During pregnancy, hormones start preparing your breast for lactation (the formation of milk in your breasts) which brings many changes to your breasts.

During the first trimester
During the first trimester your areola and nipple darken and your breasts increase in size, so you should wear a very comfortably-fitted bra. It must not be tight fitting as that will restrict blood circulation and the development of milk. The size of the lobules starts increasing, and the milk ducts expand as they fill with milk. Because of this, your breasts, particularly your nipples, will become tender against touch. You will notice this tenderness during first trimester, but it can be eased by 5-6 minutes of light massage.

During the second trimester
During the second trimester, your breasts will continue to become larger and heavier, as the duct system continues to develop and enlarge, and the lobules continue to grow. However, you will feel less tenderness and sensitivity than in the first trimester. From about the third or fourth month, your breasts begin to produce colostrum. It is the first secretion from the breasts after birth which is rich in antibodies. The blue veins under your breast skin become much more noticeable due to the increase in blood supply. As your areola and nipples grow larger, you will notice that your nipples stand out more.

During the third trimester
During the third trimester, your breasts will feel much heavier, and your nipples could start leaking colostrum by its end.

8.3   A perfect latch

The basis of breastfeeding is getting the baby to latch on well. A baby who latches on well gets milk well. A baby who latches on poorly has more difficulty getting milk, especially if the milk supply is not abundant. The milk supply is not abundant in the first few days after birth; this is normal, as nature intended, but if the baby's latch is not good, the baby has difficulty getting the milk. Even if the mother's milk production is plentiful, trying to breastfeed a baby with a poor latch is similar to giving a baby a bottle with a nipple hole that is too small—the bottle is full of milk, but the baby will not get much or will get it very slowly—so the baby sucking at the breast may spend long periods on the breast or return to the breast frequently or not be happy at the breast, all of which may convince the mother she doesn't have enough milk, which is most often not true.

If you have never breastfed a baby before, you might feel a little daunted about how you will manage this successfully. But please, put your fears aside! Following are some excellent information of different types of feeding position and guideline about how to get a perfect latch.

- Sit or lie back so that your back is supported and you feel comfortable.

- Raise your feet or your knees, if you need to.

- If you are sitting up, you could use a pillow to take the weight of your baby at first, so your forearms aren't doing all the work.

Feeding positions

The most common feeding positions include the following:

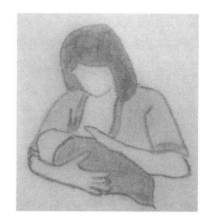

Cradle. The baby is held in the crook of elbow area of the arm on same side as breast to be used for feeding; mother supports breast with opposite hand (take C hold); baby's body is rolled in toward mother's body so they are belly-to-belly.

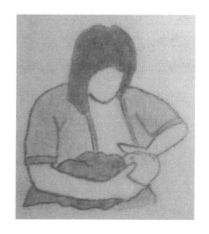

Cross-cradle. The baby's head is supported by the hand opposite the breast to be used for feeding; mother supports breast with hand (take U hold); baby is rolled in toward mother's body belly-to-belly.

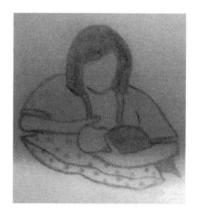

Football or clutch. Baby's head is supported by the hand on the same side as breast to be used for feeding; baby's body is supported on a pillow and tucked under the arm on the same side as breast to be used for feeding. This position also proved good to use with twin baby when you want to feed both of them at the same time.

Side-lying using modified cradle. In this position, the baby lies next to the mother so that both of their bodies are facing each other. If a pillow under your arm is uncomfortable, try placing your baby in the crook of your arm. This way, you will not be likely to roll over on the baby should you doze off. This position also keeps the baby's head at a good angle to bring baby and breast together, with the baby's head higher than his or her tummy, which can be helpful for babies who are more likely to spit up. This position is more useful in early days after delivery, especially in case of caesarian birth

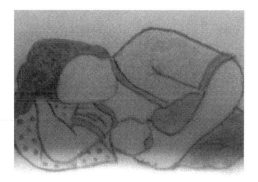

To help your baby achieve a deep latch, support your breast from underneath with your hand. A 'C-hold', with your thumb on top and your fingers underneath your breast, at least 1.5 to 2 inches behind the nipple, gives good support for the cradle or cross-cradle positions. A 'U-hold', in which you slide your hand so your thumb is on one side of the breast, your fingers on the other side and your palm near to your ribs, often used when a baby is placed in the football (clutch) position for feeding. You may not have to continue to use a C or U hold if your breasts are smaller, but mothers with larger breasts often maintain the hold throughout the feeding.

Latching on

- Sit tummy to tummy with your baby.
- Bring your baby close to your breast.
- Squash your breast slightly between your finger and the thumb so the breast is in hamburger shape and offer the baby a bite.
- Tickle the baby's lip with your nipple and wait for him or her to open wide. The baby should have a big mouthful of your breast, and his or her chin and nose should be touching your breast. Your baby's lips should be flanged outward like a trumpet or fish lips
- When the baby's mouth opens wide, bring the baby toward your breast, but not breast towards the baby.
- **Note** that the baby's mouth needs to cover your nipple + your areola + some of your breast tissue, otherwise, the milk will not flow as freely,

which can be very frustrating for your baby, and also cause the ducts to become blocked which can lead to mastitis (infected and very painful).

- When your baby's hunger is satisfied, it will naturally let go, but if it does need help to unlatch, just slide your finger into the corner of its mouth to break the suction.

If your baby is not latched on properly, you'll notice some of these signs:

- Your milk won't flow easily.
- It hurts you during breastfeeding. (When the baby is latched on properly, breastfeeding is comfortable and not painful at all.)
- Your baby sucks frantically or noisily without seeming to find a rhythm.
- Your baby doesn't seem relaxed. If the baby is getting enough milk it will calm down.
- Your baby still seems hungry even after a long feed of 40 minutes or so.
- Your baby may not gain enough weight.

8.4   Some advice on breastfeeding

Always clean your nipples and the baby's lips with warm water before and after feeding your baby. It is handy to keep some hot water ready in a thermos for this.

5-6 times a day, after a feed, gently wipe the nipple and apply ghee or castor oil to your nipple to keep it soft, moist and prevent cracks.

Be as calm and peaceful as possible while feeding.

Put a pillow on your lap to lay the baby on, so it can feed easily, whilst allowing you to sit in a good posture.

It is not advisable to feed the baby when you are lying down as it causes ear infection (the baby's sucking jaw feels pressure, which creates ear problems). If it's really necessary (because you feel discomfort from stitches or you can't sit), then you can feed the baby while lying down but only for the first 10 days.

Do not wake up your baby for a feed. It will automatically awake when it is actually hungry.

It's not advisable to feed the baby more than eight times within a 24-hour period. It's good to be punctual with feeding times to create a schedule for feeding, as this is good for the baby's hunger and health. This does not mean that you should stick to the schedule very strictly, but try to make a fair timetable; this helps you too. At night, for example, a maximum of two feeds is fair enough, so if the baby sleeps soundly from 10pm to 3am, then it's a good idea to feed it again, and then start in the morning again from 7am with a gap each time of 2 hours between feeds.

In the beginning babies can feed for around 5 minutes on each breast, and the time can then be gradually increased to 10-15 minutes on each side. There are no hard and fast rules about how long to feed the infant each time. The baby will usually feed for up to 15-20 minutes each time, and will stop sucking once it is satisfied. The baby should be fed alternatively from each breast. You could start one session with your right breast, for example, and let it empty as the last part of the milk contains a higher amount of fat which is very good for the baby. Once the right breast is empty and if the baby is still hungry, continue with your left breast or start the next session with your left breast.

Continue breastfeeding till your baby is at least 12 months old.

Breastfeeding alternative

If for some reason, it is not possible for you to breastfeed, goat's milk is the next best option, and if you can't find that, then cow's milk is another good option, but preferably organic and without any enhancements.

Preparation of Milk
Take 100ml of goat's/cow's milk + 100ml of water + 5 grains of *vavding* (*Embelia ribes*) + 1 grain of Vakumbha (careya arborea Roxb), boil and strain it. Let the mixture cool to room temperature and then it is ready for feeding your baby.

If you can't find pure and natural goat or cow milk, the last option is to use powdered milk formula available in the market that is specially prepared for babies. You can get a prescription for it from the doctor.

Feeding Chart

Here is a handy chart showing a suitable gap between the day-time feeds for your baby, as well as the suitable number of feeds per night in the age of 1 week to 1 year.

Age	Gap Between Day-time Feeds	Number of Night-time Feeds
Week 1	2 hours	2
Weeks 2-3	2 hours	2
Weeks 4-5	2 hours	1
Weeks 6-12	2 hours	1
Months 3-6	3 hours	1
Months 6-9	3 hours	1
Months 9-12	3 hours	1

You need not follow this chart very strictly. You are not meant to keep your baby waiting for a 'set feeding time' if it is hungry early. But on the other hand, do not assume that the baby's crying always means it is hungry and feeds it frequently.

There is no way to measure how much milk has been consumed. If the baby gains weight normally, sleeps well, feeds at proper intervals, has no digestion problems, is not irritable and is quiet for two-three hours after feeding, it means its needs are being adequately met.

Other reasons for crying

There are lots of other reasons for a baby to cry in addition to being hungry. Here are some very common ones. The baby might:

- feel cold or hot

- have colic pain (from having gas in its abdomen)
- have difficulty breathing, because of a blocked nose
- have an ear infection
- have an abdominal pain, because of constipation

It is only natural for a mother to wonder what is ailing her baby, but if it is crying besides feeding well and with proper intervals, it means there must be some other problem. So then you know to go through the list above and find out the real problem.

If it turns out that none of the above seems to be a problem, you may wish to consult your doctor. Sometimes though, crying is just a phase that the baby is going through. If this is the case, then your comforting touch and voice will surely help, so you can hold and rock the baby, or walk around with it and at the same time sing or talk to it. In most cases, changing the environment of the baby also helps tremendously; so take the baby outdoors in fresh air if you can or change rooms and the baby will most likely feel better in a little while.

8.5   Breast Pumping and Nursing

Who needs a pump?

You may need a pump if....

- Your baby is not nursing well (or not nursing at all). A quality pump is the best way to maintain milk supply in this situation.

- To stimulate your milk production and increase your milk supply.

- To collect milk to feed a premature baby or one who can't latch on to your breast.

- To relieve the pain and pressure of engorged breasts – though too much pumping when you're engorged can make matters worse.

- You are planning occasional separations from the baby for more than a couple of hours. Hand expression is another option.

- You plan to return to full- or part-time work and want to provide milk for the baby.

Most women express their milk using an electric or manual pump. Some women prefer to express their milk by hand but most feel that using a pump is faster and easier.

Expressed breastmilk and about storing it

Expressed breastmilk will separate when stored in the refrigerator. This can be a real shock to anyone who is not aware that this is normal. Sometimes there is a thick layer of cream or fat on top, other times a thin layer. Sometimes the milk looks lumpy, or clumpy, and sometimes it can be nearly clear toward the bottom of the bottle. All of the above are completely normal occurrences, and does not mean the milk has spoiled. Spoiled milk has a distinct sour smell.

When ready to offer to the baby, one needs only to remove from the fridge and gently swirl the milk to remix it.

The picture here shows an example of what normal breastmilk when stored in a refrigerator may look like.

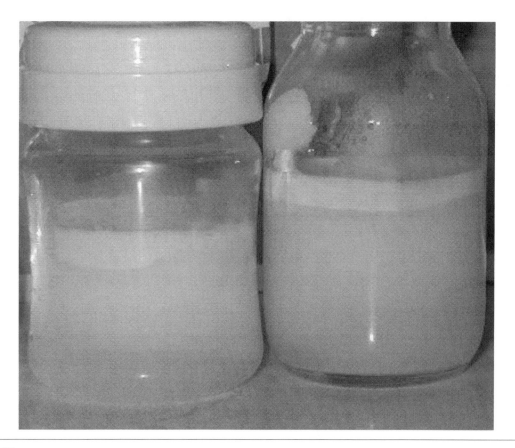

You can store expressed breastmilk in a feeding bottle and to keep it fresh in a number of ways

- At room temperature (no more than 25 degrees C), for up to six hours.
- In a cool box, with ice packs, for up to 24 hours.
- In a fridge (at four degrees C or colder), for up to five days.
- In a fridge's freezer compartment, for two weeks.

Don't be tempted to defrost or warm your breastmilk in a microwave. If you need the milk in a hurry, defrost by placing it in a bowl of warm water.

8.6   Activities that contaminate breastmilk

A number of things can contaminate your breastmilk, so here is a list of things to avoid.

- Over eating, eating too much sweets, bitter and salty food, deep-fried or stale food
- Consumption of pickles, very spicy food, and vegetables like *gavar* (cluster beans), *bhindi* (okra), cabbage, *galka* (ash gourd), *chhole* (white chickpeas), *rajma* (red kidney beans), *vaal* (field beans), as well as excess tea, coffee, alcohol or tobacco
- Sadness, anger, grief, stress and inadequate sleep
- Watching movies that create fear, thrill or deeply influence your moods
- Eating refined flour, junk food, ice-cream, etc.
- Chronic constipation also leads to less production of milk, so you need to take care of it as early on as possible

Here is the description of the characteristics of pure and healthy breastmilk by *Aacharya Sushruta*, an ancient doctor and surgeon:

Pure breastmilk is of cooling nature, thin and clean, white in color, and if by putting a drop of it in water, it dissolves easily, it is a pure and healthy milk.

Below is his description of the characteristics of breastmilk which is contaminated by *doshas*:

- If the breastmilk is put in water and floats, is bitter/astringent in taste and of slightly dark color, it is disturbed with vata dosha. This milk may cause flatulence, constipation or indigestion.
- If it is yellowish in color, sour/bitter in taste, it is disturbed by pitta dosha. This may cause loose motions, high body temperature or sweating.
- If milk sinks in water and is of sticky and heavy nature, it is disturbed by kapha dosha. This may cause frequent coughs and colds, swelling on the face or excessive salivation.

Benefits of breast feeding

There are tons of benefits of breastfeeding.

- It is a wholesome food for the baby.
- It contains all the nutrition needed by your baby.
- It helps to develop a high immunity, a sound intellect, and robust physical and mental health for your baby.
- All nutrition consumed by you can be passed to your baby via your breastmilk.
- It can reduce your stress levels and the risk of postpartum depression.
- It helps your uterus to contract and return it to its normal size quickly.
- It lowers your chances of premenopausal breast cancer and ovarian cancer, often deadly diseases that are on the rise.

8.7 Remedies to increase breastmilk

If your milk production is not at its optimal level, use these 7 remedies on daily basis. These will help to maintain the quantity and quality of your milk.

- Consume milk + rice.
- Drink milk with 1 teaspoon of *shatavari* (*Asparagus racemosus*) powder twice a day.
- Consume ghee with crystal sugar (*khada sakar*) once or twice a day.
- Boil *aerand* (castor oil plant leaves) or Neem leaves with water and strain. Then wash your breasts with this water (at an easily bearable temperature) and finally put hot leaves on the breasts, leaving them there for few minutes.
- Massage your breasts with warm oil prepared from 50 gm (1.75 ounces) of castor oil + 50 gm (1.75 ounces) of coconut oil.
- Cure your chronic constipation, if present. It interrupts the formation of milk.

- Consume 100 gm (3.5 ounces) dried grated coconut + 20-30 gm (0.75-1.0 ounces) *suva dana* (dill seeds) every day.

If your milk production decreases, here are some very good remedies to increase it again. These 5 special herbal preparations are especially effective in increasing breast milk. Pick one or two that suits you. Continue your chosen remedies until your breastmilk increases in volume again.

- Mix the herbs *piplimul* (*ganthoda* or root of the Indian long peppe), fennel (*saufa*), *ashwagandha* (Indian winter cherry), and *shatavari* in equal proportion. Drink 1 teaspoon of the mixture with milk once a day.
- Drink milk with a half teaspoon of *shatavari* (*Asparagus racemosus*) powder + half teaspoon of *vaidari kanda* (*Ipomoea digitata* or giant potato flower) powder.
- If breast milk is disturbed because of increased *vata dosha*, then mix equal quantities of *aswagandha* + *yastimadhu* + *shatavari* + *jivanti* powders. Add 2 teaspoon of this mixture to 200 gm of milk + 150 gm of water and boil it until only one cup of the preparation remains. Drink this after you've added 2 teaspoons of castor oil to it. Continue having 1 cup a day of this preparation until your breastmilk increases.
- Mix equal quantities of *pipali* (Indian long pepper) + *suthi* (dry ginger powder) + *harde* (*Terminalia chebula*) powder. Mix 3 gm of this mixture with *gud* (jaggery) + ghee, and consume this preparation twice a day for two months.
- Chew 4-5 seeds of *Kamal kakadi* (lotus seed). It is a black shield herb with white portion in it. Break the shield and chew well the white portion of the herb.

8.8   When and how to stop breastfeeding (weaning)

It's best to give your baby nothing but breastmilk for the first six months of its life. After that, you can start to introduce different liquid foods mentioned in the section, *Baby's Diet* in Chapter 10 *Baby Care* as well as continue breastmilk. Naturally the question arises about when it's the right time to wean your baby i.e. to stop breastfeeding.

Generally, at the age of 9-10 months, it's the right time to start reducing the frequency of the breastfeeds. Often by this age babies themselves give up breastfeeding, which can be an emotional experience both for you and your baby, but if you go step by step then it could be done with ease.

Once you decide to stop breastfeeding, don't do it abruptly as that's not good for either of you. Take 2-3 months to reduce the frequency of breastfeeds so your baby can adjust. Weaning may take longer if you try before your baby is ready. There is no fixed rule about how much time your baby will take to stop breastfeeding, as some take 10-15 days and some take 4-5 months, but by the age of 12-16 months your baby should be weaned off from your breast.

Remember though that even after weaning your baby, it will still require at least 1-2 glasses of cow's or goat's milk per day as part of its diet.

....

So this now concludes the chapter on breastfeeding, in which you have learned how to breastfeed, and how to look after yourself so that your milk supply is healthy and plentiful. You will enjoy the efficiency and comfort of breastfeeding your baby, at the same time knowing that this is the best possible thing for your baby you can do.

In the next chapter, we turn to the subject of how to take best care for yourself – the mother, during the period after your baby is born.

Care of the Mother

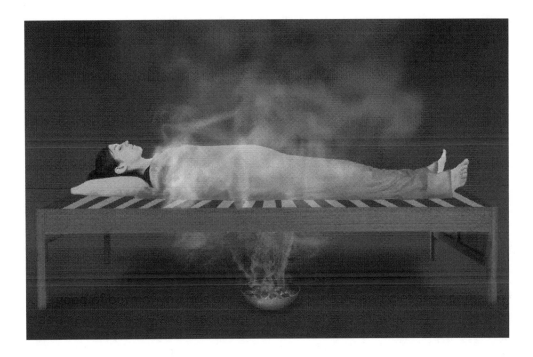

This chapter is about the care of the mother in the short time period after delivery. She is referred to as *Sutika* for 45 days after delivery.

For the good of both of you, it's obvious that your care and diet are optimal in the time as a new mother – and that is what this chapter is all about!

There are two parts to this chapter and they cover the care of the new mother and also her diet.

9.1 Care of the new mother

The postpartum (just after the birth) period is a time for deep rest and rejuvenation for the new mother. This is the time when there are high chances of *vata* imbalance in the body. Ayurveda describes some essential activities which every new mother should follow, in order to expel an excess *vata* imbalance, aid digestion, get back into shape and regain the strength after undergoing an extreme exertion during labor. If the new mother does not take care of herself properly, it is not just herself but also her precious newborn who will suffer.

So ... Here are some essential activities for you to be healthier, fitter and quickly get back into shape again.

Massage

Three or five days after normal delivery, have a massage with warm oil. This practice should be continued for a minimum of 45 days. It is better if you can continue it for up to 3 months. If possible, massage should be done on the floor on a single blanket or mat, as a hard surface is good for your back and helps to get your tummy back into shape quickly. After a C-section too, you can start massage from the fifth day, but massage your back in a sitting position. Don't massage your tummy. As soon as the doctor allows you to lie down on your abs, you can start using the normal massage position on the floor.

You'll find that the massage alleviates fatigue and pain. It also prevents you from cold and infection. It helps to correct your *vata* imbalance, aids your digestive system and tones up your body. Rather than simply using til oil, it is better to prepare some special oil.

Oil Preparation

- Take 100 gm (3½ ounces) of *til* (sesame)oil + 10 gm (⅓ ounce) of *vaja* (*calamus* or sweet flag) + 10 gm (⅓ ounce) of *malkangani* (*celastrus paniculatus*) and heat it properly. Then strain it and the oil is ready to use. If you wish, *suthi* (dried ginger powder) also can be added.
- *Balaswagandhadi taila* (an Ayurvedic medicated oil) or *ksheera bala taila* (a traditional Ayurvedic massage oil) can be used as well. These provide strength to your ligaments, muscles, tendons and joints. They will both be effective in relaxing your body. It is really available in the market.

Bath

You'll find that it is always good to take bath with hot water, or warm water in summer. During the bath stay out of any direct breeze. A good time for bathing is in the afternoon, or after sunrise when air is a bit warm. Instead of using soap, use a specially prepared *Ubtan* (organic herbal and grain paste used as soap). It is also better to use specially prepared bath water, instead of plain water.

Ubtan

Each of these *ubtans* will smooth and brighten your skin, prevent stretch marks, and soothe your mind with its fragrance.

- *Chana* (chickpea flour) + milk cream works well.
- *Chana* (chickpea flour) + *masoor dal flour* (split red lentil flour) + *jav* flour (oatmeal) also works well.

Adding some herbs like turmeric, *nagarmotha* (*Cyperus rotundus)*, sandalwood or *suganthi vado* (Vetiveria Zizanioides) to either of these preparations is more beneficial.

Bath water

- Boil a few *nirgundi* leaves *(Vitex negundo)* + castor oil leaves + neem leaves in 2-3 liters (4.25-6 pints) of water and add this preparation to your hot bath water. These herbs are anti-infective, anti-viral and *vata* purifiers.
- To pamper yourself even more you can make an aroma bath, by adding a few drops of aroma oil to hot water. Jasmine is good for preventing postnatal depression. Eucalyptus helps to reduce cold and congestion in your chest. Rosemary and lavender have soothing effects.

Hot dry fomentation

The next very essential activity is to have a hot dry fomentation. Customarily, a traditional *khaat* (cot), made from woven ropes and covered with thin cotton cloth. The new mother lies down on this wearing thin clothes. Charcoal and cow dung cakes are put in a big pan or vessel (*choki*), and lit with fire. Once the fire has died down and the embers are producing an even regular heat, the vessel is put under the *khaat* and the new mother basks in the scented, hot dry fomentation for about 15-30 minutes.

The mother should feel the heat of the fomentation all over her body, especially on her waist and back. This hot dry fomentation helps to pacify *vata* and strengthen the body. It prevents back pain, flatulence, joint pain and gas formation in the abdomen.

In winter one can do this at any time of the day, but generally people prefer to take it after a bath. You can also sprinkle *ajwain* (caraway seeds) on the charcoal. In summer it is more convenient to take the fomentation at night when it is a bit cooler.

If it is not possible for you to take a hot dry fomentation with a *khaat*, you could use an electric hot-pad instead, but using a *khaat* is the best.

You can continue this practice for 45 days after your delivery, and then can reduce it to every second day, and finally to 2-3 days a week.

Abdominal Belt

As mentioned previously in Chapter 6, the abdominal belt should be tied just after your delivery and should not be removed any time except when bathing. It helps your abdominal muscles and uterus to return to their shape and also supports your back. It should be used for 45 days after your delivery.

Covering the Ears

As mentioned previously in Chapter 6, your ears should be covered with a small ball of cotton and also a scarf just after labor to keep them warm and out of any breeze or draughts. This should continue for 45 days after your delivery too.

9.2   Diet for the new mother

The reason for consuming the below mentioned diet is to strengthen your body, help your uterus return to its original condition and health, expel excess *vata* (which is naturally generated after birth) and also to increase your breast milk.

There are two parts to this diet. The first part contains three special preparations for you to consume each day. The second part contains the sort of foods that you would normally consider eating for lunch and dinner. The ones listed here have been especially selected as they are highly beneficial for you throughout your entire period as a new mother.

Preparations

1. Add 10 gm (0.35 ounce) of *Suva* (dill seed) + 5 gm (0.17 ounce) of *methi* (fenugreek seed) to 1 liter (2 pints) of water and boil it till only 250 ml (½ pint) remains, then add 10 gm (⅓ ounce) of honey. Drink this decoction in the morning on an empty stomach.

   Suva expels excess *vata* from the stomach, increases digestive fire, and also helps cleanse the uterus.

   Methi strengthens the joints, so it helps your back and knees, also strengthens all the muscles of your body. It also expels *vata*.

2. After consuming above, gulp down *heerabol* (Commiphora myrrha) herb, quantity the size of a *kala chana* (chickpea), while taking care that it doesn't touch your teeth.

   Heerabol is anti-inflammatory, antimicrobial and antiseptic, and treats colds, coughs, diarrhea, flatulence and hemorrhoids. It gives excellent results for infections of uterus and vagina, and is also very effective for menstrual pains, amenorrhea, dysmenorrhea and uterine tumors. In addition to that, it is also used for the treatment of gum problems like sore throat, gum sores, and toothache.

3. After consuming above have *raab* – (see *Recipe* section in Chapter 12 – Miscellaneous.)

For Days 1-5: Consume Preparations 1, 2 & 3 for the first 5 days after delivery.

For Days 6-45: Stop Preparation 1 and continue with Preparations 2 & 3 for days 6-45.

Dishes and foods for you to consume

This section contains the food that you will consume. There are dishes to choose for your meals, *dals* (pulses), veggies, spices, some herbal preparations, plus some mouth fresheners, and specially prepared water to drink every day.

- **Dishes**

  Following is the list of items which can be part of your lunch or dinner and they can be consumed on a daily basis to improve your health.

  - *sheera* (a traditional Indian sweet made with semolina) – see *Recipe* section in Chapter 12.
  - *chapati* (Indian bread)
  - *bhakhari* (Indian bread)
  - *rotala* (Indian bread made from millet)
  - *raab* (a special liquid preparation) – see *Recipe* section in Chapter 12.
  - *methi ladoo* and *dink ladoo* (edible gum ladoo). These are sweet dishes. See *Recipe* section in Chapter 12.
  - lentil soup
  - vegetable soup
  - ghee (home-made butter)
  - buttermilk
  - *paneer* (cottage cheese)
  - rice
  - katlu/shobhagya suthi paak (a traditional Ayurvedic formulation)
  - *khichdi* (a traditional rice and lentil dish)
  - *bajri thepla* (Indian millet bread)

- ***Dal* (pulses)**

  Mung and *mung dal* (green and yellow lentils) are the best to have regularly, while *tur dal* (pigeon peas) and *kulath dal* (horse gram) are good to have occasionally.

- **Veggies**

  These vegetables are suitable for you to include in your lunch or dinner every day.

dudhi (bottle gourd)	*turiya* (ridge gourd)
tinda (ivy gourds)	*methi* (fenugreek) leaves
parval (*trichosanthes anguina*)	Garlic and onion

tandalja bhaji (amaranthus)	bengan (brinjal)
karela (bitter gourd)	palak (spinach)

- **Some essential spices**

  All these spices are very important and you should use them frequently in different types of food preparations. Ayurveda puts a big emphasis on spices because they purify *vata*, increase digestive fire, increase breast milk, purify blood and strengthen the body.

taj (cinnamon)	*jeera* (cumin seeds)	*pudina* (mint)
dry coconut	*tamal patra* (bay leaf)	*tulsi* (basil)
ajwain (celery seeds)	coriander leaves	neem leaves
hing (asafetida)	chilly	*suva* (dill seed)
black pepper	ginger and dried ginger	*haldi* (turmeric)

- **Mouth Freshener**

  You can use following ingredients as part of your mouth freshener:

  Soph (fennel seed), *amla* (Indian gooseberry), *til* (sesame seed), *ajwain* (celery seed) and *suva* (dill seed).

- **Herbal Preparations**
  - **Dashamoola tea**

    This tea soothes *vata* in your pelvic region, which is very important for proper rejuvenation!

    Boil 2 cups of water + 2 teaspoons of *dashamoola* powder (ready available in the market). Boil down to ½ cup, and take ¼ cup warm, in morning and evening. Refrigerate the unused portion and rewarm. Make fresh daily.

    OR

  - **Dashmoolarishta**

    This is available in the market and you can have 2 teaspoon of syrup + 2 teaspoon of water twice a day after each meal.

o **Shatavari** *(Asparagus racemosus* powder*)*

Consume 1 teaspoon of *shatavari* powder + milk or ghee every day. It is very good for lactation, as well as strength and hormonal balance.

(Note: Take Shatavari and either of Dashamoola tea or Dashmoolarishta)

- **Drinking water for daily use**

You should drink any of the following drinking water preparations rather than normal water.

o **Hot drinking water 1**

Boil 2 quarts (2 liters) of water + ½ teaspoon each of fennel and fenugreek seeds for 10 minutes. Keep in a thermos and drink warm throughout the day. Refrigerate unused portion and rewarm. Make fresh daily.

It supports your hydration, lactation, digestion and rejuvenation.

o **Hot drinking water 2**

Take 2 quarts (2 liters) of water + 4-5 pieces of *vakumba* (*Careya arborea*) and 10-15 grain of *vavding* (*embelia ribes*). Boil and strain, and keep in a thermos so you can drink it warm throughout the day.

It aids your digestive system and corrects gas formation in your abdomen.

A sample daily regime

To give you an idea of how this might work in practice, here is a sample daily regime for you to look at.

1. In the morning have Preparations 1, 2 and 3.
2. Mix equal quantities of *suva* (dill seeds) + dry grated coconut + *til* (sesame seeds) + finely chopped *kharek* (dried dates). Consume 50 gm (about 1.75 ounces) of the mixture regularly throughout the whole day.
3. For lunch you can have *sheera*, chapati, *rotala*, *thepla*, *puri*, and any of the veggies from the list, rice and dal.

4. For snacks between 4 to 5 pm have lentil or veggie soup or *raab* (see *Recipe* section in Chapter 12).
5. For dinner you can have *khichdi, bajri thepla, rotalo* etc.
6. Use the hot water preparations above as your drinking water.
7. Drink 1 cup milk + *satavari* (*Asparagus racemosus*) powder once a day.
8. You can have buttermilk after 12 days post-delivery, but consume it before 3 pm. Add ½ teaspoon of *piplimool* (Indian long pepper) powder to 1 glass of buttermilk. It increases digestive fire and reduces fat from the tummy.
9. If you are feeling tired and uneasy, you can consume *jaggery* water. Pepper, ginger and *chitraka* (*Plumbago zeylanica*) can also be added for flavor.
10. After delivery for 45 days, Ayurveda advises you take about 5-10 ml (⅙-⅓ ounces) of sesame oil or ghee twice a day. If you can't face consuming raw ghee, you can mix it with 2-3 gm (about 0.1 ounces) of herbal powder that is made by combining various ingredients such as ginger, *chavya chaba* (Balinese long pepper) and *chitraka* (*plumbago zeylanica*). This helps to relax your body.

....

So this now concludes the chapter about caring for yourself as a new mother (*sutika*). These activities plus the diet provide the best support for your health during this time, as well as provide remedies for the common problems that generally occur.

And of course, if you are receiving the best care possible, you are in the best position for giving your precious baby the best possible care too so it can thrive in its new life! And care of the baby is the subject for the next chapter!

Baby Care

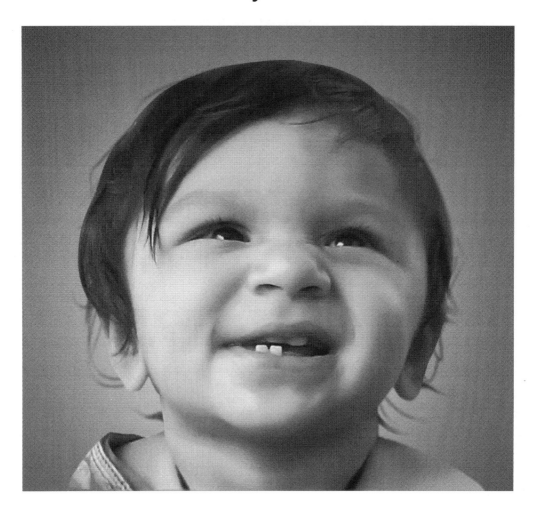

Till now we have discussed the care of your darling baby just after delivery. Now we will discuss some essential day to day activities and foods that are recommended by Ayurveda to improve your baby's health and development, especially over the first three years. It provides a healthy foundation, which is essential as the baby grows.

You'll also find discussions on Ayurvedic methods that you can use to work out on the complaints your baby might be suffering from.

10.1   Care of the Baby

Now that you've got your baby home, you might be wondering what you actually need to do each day to care for it! This section discusses a series of lovely activities that you can carry out daily with your baby. You'll find that they are enjoyable things to do with your baby, and the baby will enjoy them too.

Massage

Before bath, massage your baby gently with a specially prepared oil. Oil massage keeps the baby's skin soft and supple, opens up the pores in the skin, enhances blood circulation, and encourages its bones to be stronger and well-shaped. Oil massage also aids digestion, relieves colic, eases tension, regulates breathing and spurs growth.

When massaging your baby be gentle and soft, as applying pressure to the baby's body, or rubbing its skin forcefully could cause injury. Massage the baby playfully and lovingly.

Preparation of oil

- You'll need 100 gm of *amla*(dried Indian gooseberry) + 2.5 gm of *vaja* (calamus root/sweet flag) + 10 gm of rose petals + 5 gm of *kapoor kachli* (*Hedychium spicatum* or spiked ginger lily) + 5 gm of henna leaves + 5 gm of Sugandhi Vado (Vetiveria Zizanioides). Grind all of these with a little water and to make a pulpy paste. Add the paste to 400 gm of *til oil* (sesame oil). Boil the mixture over a low flame till the paste turns light red in color, then strain it. This oil can be used to massage the baby's body and head and also for putting some drops in the baby's ears.
- You can also use *til* oil + coconut oil + almond oil OR just coconut oil OR pure ghee to massage the baby as these all work very well too.

Precaution

- Make sure that the room is warm, especially in winter.
- Put some cream on your hands and rub them together so they will be soft and warm before starting.
- Your nails should be properly trimmed.

How to Massage the Baby

Ayurveda says that you should start the massage by applying a good quantity of oil to the baby's fontanel (crown chakra) so it gets absorbed. Then massage should be done in upwards direction, starting with the soles of the feet, and then the legs, thighs, stomach, chest, palms, hands, shoulders, face, hips, back, neck and finally the head. Massage very gently in a circular clockwise movement.

After the massage, let the oil soak into the baby's body, so that after about half an hour later you can bathe the baby. During this time, it is also good to take the baby in soft sunlight near a window, but without it coming into direct contact with any breeze or draught.

Baby Bath

Between 10am to 3pm is a good time to bath the baby, as there is less humidity or cold at this time, especially in winter. If this is not possible, adjust the room temperature.

The water used to bathe the baby should be neither too hot nor too cold. Do not use soap but use one of the following:

- *besan* (chickpea flour) mixed with *malai* (the cream) or with milk.
- *Ubbattan* (see preparation below).

Preparation of Ubbattan

Take 50gm of *besan* (chickpea flour) + 5gm of *haldi* (turmeric) + 5gm of *amla* (Indian gooseberry) powder + 2.5 gm of *shikakai* (*Acacia concinna*) powder. Mix all these finely ground powders with a little oil and your *ubbattan* is ready to use. If you wish, you can also add sandalwood powder to it.

When you have gently dried your baby after bath, put 2 drops of the specially prepared oil in the baby's ears and rub gently so it can penetrate deep inside.

Dhoop

Dhoop means to give smoke to the baby and this is done after the baby has bathed.

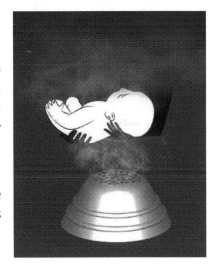

The traditional method of making *dhoop* is to light some charcoal or dried cow dung, and once it starts smoking, expose the baby to the smoke. You can also add *ajwain* (caraway seeds) and *guggal* (the sticky gum from myrrh trees) to the *dhoop* mixture.

You must check the temperature of the smoke carefully, felt by the baby, to make sure it does not feel very hot.

It is also advisable to cover the dhoop pan with a large sieve, so the baby is not directly exposed to the heat, but still allows the smoke to reach all parts of the baby's body –its head, ears, back, anus and genitals. You can administer dhoop daily till the baby is 6-8 months old, but after that it is difficult to hold the baby for it.

Dhoop prevents coughs, colds, congestion of *kapha* (mucus) in the lungs, keeps the body temperature correct after a bath, and checks humidity in the baby's body. It also works as a disinfectant if cow dung or neem (*Azadirachta indica*) leaves are added to it.

After *dhoop* the baby is ready to be dressed.

Clothing

Dress your baby with comfortable cotton clothes. They should be washed properly and dried. According to Ayurveda, these clothes should also be given *dhoop*. It is advisable not to use diapers or at least, minimize their use, as diapers always keep the genital area moist, which creates infection and sagging skin, and also creates rashes.

Urination and Defecation

Babies first urinate within 4-5 hours after birth and defecate within 4-6 hours after birth. If 10-12 hours passed and the baby has still not urinated, then you must check with the doctor. For a baby boy, there is a possibility that the penis is blocked by a toxic particle, which should be cleaned out.

The same happens with defecation. If the baby has not passed stool within 4-6 hours after birth, it should be consulted by the doctor for an internal problem. But if the baby doesn't having any internal problems and still doesn't pass a stool, you can give it 10 drops of castor oil with the *gadthuthi* (Please refer to the section, *Gadthuthi* in Chapter 6) or with breast milk, and within 2 hours of that the baby should defecate.

Generally, babies up to 2 months urinate every 2-3 hours and defecate every 4-5 hours. As the baby grows these intervals increase. After 3 months, it is 3-4 hours for urination and 6-8 hours for defection. These intervals may vary according to season as well as the baby's constitution.

The proper stool for a breastfed baby is yellow in color, soft and odorless. If the baby suffers from diarrhea while you are fully breastfeeding it, then it is advisable for you to change your diet to a *sattvik* one. If the stool is greenish colored and accompanied by watery substance, it means the baby is suffering from indigestion which requires correction. (Please refer to the *'Know the Symptoms'* section below.)

Baby's Cradle

Using a cradle for a sleeping baby is a great tradition because the slow and rhythmic motion of the rocking cradle, puts the baby to sleep and also creates a lovely and cozy feeling. Be careful though not to rock the cradle too fast and not to rock it once baby is asleep.

Two types of cradle are available: one that keeps the back of the baby straight, and one that gives a slight curve to the back (spine). Both types are absolutely fine.

10.2 Balguti/Ghasaro (Bitters)

Balguti/Ghasaro is made by grinding a few particular herbs with mother's milk or even water on a specially made grinding stone. It is a common tradition to feed an infant with *Balguti* every day, to keep it fit and healthy, and to prevent and cure common diseases.

Balguti helps to ensure proper digestion, bowel movement and boost the immune system. It prevents and cures cold, cough, fever, constipation, diarrhea, vomiting and so on. It also helps the baby to gain good weight and have sound sleep. *Balguti* also contains some herbs which sharpens the mind and increases life span.

Balguti should be started when the baby is 15 days old and continued until it is fifteen months old.

Herbs in Balguti

If the baby is fit and well, not all herbs are required in *Balguti,* but a few of them work extremely well and are so safe enough to be used on a daily basis. Following are lists of herbs which should be used in a daily basis. These ones help the baby to gain weight, increase its digestive capacity, have a glowing skin and memory as well as aid constipation and gas.

Dosage

When the baby is 15 days old, grind each herb on grinding stone in a circle the size of 1 rupee coin for twice in clockwise direction.

When it is 1 month old, grind for 3-4 times. As the age increases, increase grinding iterations. Take 7-8 iterations at the age of 6 months.

Herbs for Daily Use in Balguti

Herb	Effect
Badam (almond)	This is nutritious and beneficial for the brain. It also promotes intelligence and strengthens *dhatus.*

Haldi (turmeric)	This balances *kapha-vata*. It purifies blood, gives a glow to the skin, improves liver function and helps in skin problems.
Harde (chebula Terminalia)	This stimulates the appetite and liver function. It removes constipation, gas and worms. It also improves digestion and nourishes the *dhatu*. If the baby has a tendency towards constipation or gas, you should increase the proportion of *harde* in the *Balguti*.
Kakach (Pongamia glabra)	This is a black shelled nut containing a white portion. Only use the white portion. It removes worms, fever and gas. It is nutritive and digestive. This is used for skin ailments and is valued as an antiseptic and astringent. It is bitter, a blood purifier, pungent and tonic, and useful in bronchitis and whooping cough also.
Yastimadhu (Glycyrrhiza glabra)	This is of a cooling nature and it expels excess *pitta-vata*. It is nutritive for the baby, improves voice quality and brings luster to the skin. It also removes constipation, cough, and breathing difficulties due to *kapha*(phlegm) accumulated in the chest.
Ashwagandha (Withania Somnifera)	It increases strength, immune system and health. It has rejuvenating properties and nourishes *shukra dhatu* (male semen and female egg).
Kharek (dried dates)	This balances *vata, pitta* and is of a cooling nature. It improves strength of body and bones. It is very nourishing for the child.

Other herbs can be added to the *Balguti* depending on the baby's health requirement. For example:

- For coughs and colds – you can add *pimpli* (long pepper), *sunthi* (dry ginger), *kakadshing* (wax tree).
- For frequent gas formation - you can add *suva* (dill), *vavding* (Embelia ribes), *sanchar* (black salt), *sunthi* (dry ginger).

- For worms - you can add *vavding* (Embelia ribes), *harde* , a few drops of castor oil and *indrajav* (*Holarrhena pubescens*).
- For loose motions - you can add *ativisa* (Aconitum heterophyllum).

Following is the list of the herbs which can be used as per requirement to treat special condition.

Herbs for Special Medicinal Uses

Herb	Effect
Indrajav (*Holarrhena pubescens*)	This improves digestion, increases digestive fire and removes gas, and fever.
Vavding (Embelia ribes)	This cleans the body and removes heat and gas. It aids digestion and purifies the blood.
Suva(dill)	This works excellently on gas and improves appetite and digestion.
Tulsi(*Ocimum tenuiflorum* or basil)	This aids the digestive processes and controls fever. It helps to alleviate pain in the abdomen, vomiting or diarrhea. It should be used in limited quantity, and ground on the grinding stone for only a maximum of 4-5 rounds.
Mango guttli (mango kernals)	This is of cooling nature. It expels excess heat, helps in dysentery, diarrhea, colitis and so on.
Sanchad (black salt)	This is of a cooling nature. It removes indigestion, abdominal pain and works excellently for gas.
Kadu	This removes indigestion and fever.

Kakadshingi (*Rhus succedaneaee*)	This reduces *kapha* and *vata*. It aids coughs, hiccoughs, and lung problems.
Sunthi (dry ginger)	This helps the digestive process, loose motions, removes gas, reduces coughs and colds, and binds the stool properly.
Pimpli/ piplimool (long pepper)	This is mainly used for respiratory and digestive system problems. If the child has a tendency to frequent coughs, colds, or appetite loss, it works well. It is also good for indigestion.
nagarmotha (*Cyperus rotundus*)	This is cooling in nature and facilitates the digestive process. It is very helpful for loose motions. It also works as a brain tonic.
Ativisa (*Aconitum heterophyllum*)	This aids the digestive process. It cures fever, vomiting, diarrhea and colic. But it should not be used no a daily basis but only to treat these particular problems.

10.3 Baby's Diet

The main concept in Ayurveda as far as diet and nutrition are concerned is *agni* (fire). *Agni* is usually translated as "enzymes" and indicates our capacity for digestion. In other words, the *agni* of a person tells us how best the person is able to digest. To digest means to assimilate nutrients and evacuate the waste, so as a result, *agni* also refers to that digestive function that distinguishes between the nutritive and non-nutritive (waste) components of food.

Babies are born with an *agni* potential, but their *agni* is not functioning at birth. Thus, all dietary rules for babies are based on what we can do to activate the baby's *agni* successfully. A failure to start the correct functioning of *agni* leads to a number of health problems, and eventual food sensitivities and food allergies. Classic examples of these kinds of problems are colic pain, diarrhea and skin rashes such as eczema.

Ayurveda advises that a baby should be breast fed for at least six months, and up to one or two years. During the period of breastfeeding any treatments for the baby are given to the mother, but once the baby is given other food as well, then both the mother and the baby are treated. When the baby is exclusively on food, then the baby alone is treated.

1 to 6 months

The baby should be fed exclusively on breast milk at this time, or at least for the first 4 months.

6 to 12 months

The baby can slowly be introduced to liquid and semi-liquid food.

According to Ayurveda at the *Annaprashan Sanskar* (ceremony for the child's first feeding of solid food), when the child is in its sixth month, it should be fed a very small quantity of s*emolina kheer* (semolina porridge) for the very first time on an auspicious day. From this month you can add cooked rice water, mung dal in liquid form, vegetable soup, fruit juice, *raagi kheer* (finger millet porridge), raab (See Recipe section in Chapter 12) and *bhaidku* (spicy porridge- check ch-12), as they are all good options.

The classic texts of Ayurveda indicate that children should have cereals and grains as their first food because they build tissue strength. They are also easy to digest for the baby's budding *agni*. Cereals should be the child's main food until the age of 8-10 years. Fruit is basically cleansing and cooling in nature, although a few exceptions exist, and can be useful if the child tends towards hard stools and constipation. However according to Ayurveda, fruit does not build strength, so it should not be used as the child's main food, but rather as a supplement.

All food should be introduced into the baby's diet very gradually. The basic concept is that *agni* needs time to adapt to each food in order to digest it. Therefore, the rule is to introduce one new food at a time. Keep presenting this food for some time until you are sure the child can digest it (that is, there is no colic or other reaction), and then introduce the next new food. For example, first start with cooked rice water for 10-15 days and if the baby is fine with this, then add other food like fruit juice, and again wait for 10-15 days to introduce another new food.

1 to 2 years

After the first year, the amount of liquid in the child's diet can be gradually reduced. You can introduce soft cooked rice instead of rice water, steamed mashed apple instead of apple juice and so on.

During this time, you can introduce *khichdi* (a rice + lentil dish), *dal and rice (lentils + rice dish)*, *sheera* (check recipe in ch-12), *upma* (a thick porridge of dry roasted semolina), *curd and rice*, *dalia* (a cracked wheat + vegetables dish). For fruits, you can introduce mashed banana, papaya, pear and mango. Among vegetables, you can introduce *dudhi* (bottle gourd), carrots, *parval* (Pointed gourd), *methi* (fenugreek leaves), tomatoes, spinach and beetroot, all of which need to be overly cooked and mashed. For the flavor add grated fresh coconut, lemon, coriander or a tiny amount of chili powder. Later on you can also start dates, raisins and figs.

2 years onwards

Now the child will have all its teeth so it can be introduced to solid food. The child's diet should include a complete meal consisting of chapati, vegetables, dal, rice, buttermilk, etc.

Do and Don'ts
- Don't introduce sugar to your baby till it is 1 year old, and after that use *mishri* (candy sugar) or *jaggery* or honey for sweetness instead of white sugar.
- Even if your child has started solid food, still give it milk on a daily basis. It's highly nutritious.
- Avoid giving food that is not easy to digest, such as *chavali* (yard long beans), *rajma* (kidney beans), *chhole* (chickpeas), cheese, peas and sprouts, sour fruits like orange, pineapple, guava, custard apple and strawberry at least for 2 years.
- Strictly avoid giving your child white flour and bakery preparations like cakes, biscuits and chocolate.

- Avoid giving your child fried food, tinned and junk food.
- Never mix fruits with milk.
- Feed more of calcium and protein rich foods.
- Eat dinner by 7 to 8 pm.

10.4   Know the Symptoms

According to Ayurveda you can detect a problem your baby suffers just by inspecting its stool, urine, etc. As the baby is so small it can't tell you what is wrong, so it will just cry, cry and cry, which of course, will make you tense and at a loss about what to do. But with the help of Ayurveda, this is no longer a problem. You just note the symptoms and most probably you will be able to work out what the problem is.

- If your baby is breastfed and frequently vomits, it is suffering from indigestion.
  Treatment:
  o You must correct your diet, by eating *sattvik* food as described in the *sutika* diet (in Chapter 9) and avoid contra-indicated food.
  o If the baby is older than six months, then it should not be given milk or any other food but just warm water and *osaman* (mung water) with *haldi* (turmeric) and salt. Once it recovers, gradually introduce *sattvik* food.

- Check your baby's tongue. If it appears white coated with embossed dots on it, it is suffering from indigestion, so use the treatment above.

- If the baby passes a sticky stool or if it defecates frequently with only minor amounts of stool, it is suffering from dysentery.
  Treatment:
  o You must exclude heavy, sweet and spicy food from your diet.

- If your baby frequently touches its genitals or anus and has the urge to scratch, or if it clenches its teeth, it has worms in its stomach. Puffiness on the upper lip is also a symptom of this.
  Treatment:
  o ¼ teaspoon castor oil + 60 drops of *suva*(dill seed)water+ ¼ teaspoon of honey.
  o Increase the amount of herbs Kakach, Vavding , Harde and indrajav in Balguti.

- If the baby's urine leaves light blue stains after drying ,the baby is not digesting the food properly; calcium and phosphorus are being passes in the urine.
  Treatment: Please consult a doctor.

- If the baby's stool is sticky and blackish colored, it has *vata* imbalance.
  Treatment:
  In *Balguti* add½ teaspoon of *harde* + 1 pinch of *sanchar* (black salt) + 1 pinch of *ajwain*(caraway) powder. This may lead to 2-3 bowel movements. This quantity is for a 1-1½ year old child, but reduces it if the child is younger.

- If the baby's stool is of white colored, it has digestion problems.
  Treatment:
  o To increase digestive fire make the following preparation. Soak 10gm of kadiyatu (Andrographis paniculata) in 100ml of water overnight, strain the water, and give 1 teaspoon of water thrice a day.

- If the baby's stool smells badly, or its mouth has an odor, and at the same time it does not get properly hungry and avoids food, it means the baby is constipated.
  Treatment:
  o Don't force the baby to eat, but let it eat or feed whenever it desires.
  o Give castor oil or *harde* powder mixed with breastmilk or water to cure constipation. Once the constipation is cleared, the baby will start eating properly again.

- If the baby cries without reason, and putting your hand on its stomach makes it cry more, but pampering its lower abdomen seems to make it feel better, it means the baby has gas.
  Treatment:
  o Boil 1-2 pinches of *ajwain* (celery powder) in 1 cup of milk. Strain it and give to the baby.
  o You can also massage the baby's lower abdomen with castor oil in a downward direction.

- If the baby has a pain or an infection in its ear, it will cry and once you carry it on your shoulder, it will try to press its ear against your shoulder.
  Treatment: Consult a doctor.

- The baby may also cry at night if its nasal passage gets blocked.
  Treatment:
  o You can use nasal drops.
  o Slightly elevate the baby's head while it sleeps.

o   Use eucalyptus oil on its clothes and bed.

10.5   Remedies for Common Problems

If the child is raised according to Ayurvedic principles, there are fewer chances of it getting ill. Still Ayurveda prescribes some very safe and gentle remedies for the common problems that babies suffer. The intention of Ayurveda is to avoid strong medicines or antibiotics, but if the child using these remedies does not improve, you must consult a good Ayurvedic doctor. The mother also should watch her diet if the child is breastfeeding, and even take the appropriate herbs so she can cure her baby through the breast milk.

Abdominal Pain and Gas

These are very common problems, and nearly all babies and infants suffer from them. Now the question is how do you know if the baby is suffering from abdominal pain or colic? For that, please refer to the previous section, *'Know the Symptoms'*.

- In the *Balguti* grind a little more *harde*, *sanchad* (black salt), *kakach, a*nd *vavding*.
- Prepare a paste of *hing* (asafetida) with hot water and apply it on the baby's lower abdomen.
- Massage lukewarm castor oil on the baby's lower abdomen with downward movements.
- Put a pad or handkerchief on a pan to heat it, and, after it is warm enough, but not too hot, place it on the baby's abdomen for some instant relief.
- Dill water works excellently for the baby.
- The mother should eat *ajwain* (celery seeds), *sindhav* (rock salt), and *suva* (dill seeds).

Constipation

This is the second most common problem that babies suffer from. We discussed earlier in the section, *'Know the Symptoms'* that newborns defecate every 4-5 hours, and once the baby's digestive system matures, the frequency reduces to once or twice a day.

- *'Harde'* works excellent to cure constipation, so increase its portion in the *Balguti*.
- The baby who is frequently constipated can also be given a few drops of castor oil once every 15 days.
- Garmado/amaltas (*Cassia fistula* OR Golden shower tree) fruit pulp also works excellently. Soak about 50 grams of fruit pulp in water overnight. Strain and use it with about 25 grams of jaggery.
- Soak 10-15 raisins in warm water for 10-15 minute, strain and give the water to the baby.
- You can also apply castor oil to the baby's anus area.

Vomiting

Many times babies vomit after feeding, but if that happens only once in a while it is absolutely normal. But if the frequency of vomiting is higher, and you feel that your baby is not able to digest milk and gets weaker day by day, it requires treatment.

- If the symptoms are frequent then grind *kapoor kachli* (Hedychium Spicatum) 3-4 times with water, add 2 drops of honey and give it to the baby.
- Mix equal quantities of powders of *kakadshingi* + *piplimool* + *ativisa*. Take a small portion of this mixture, add honey to it and make a paste and give to the baby.

Worms or Reduced Appetite

Worms normally cause a reduced appetite.
- Mix 2 pinches of *vavding* powder with 1 teaspoon of honey. This quantity can be given to the baby all at once, or it can be split in halves and used for two serves during the day.
- Mix 5-6 drops of castor oil + 60 drops of dill water (*suva* water) + honey to the baby once in a day.
- Please refer to Chapter 5, 'All about Acupressure in Pregnancy' as well.

Cough and Cold

- Mix ½ teaspoon of ginger juice + ½ teaspoon of honey and give to a 2 years old child twice a day. Reduce the quantity if the child is younger than that; it may cause 2-3 bowel movements.

- Mix ⅛-¼ teaspoon of *sitopaladi* (an Ayurvedic medicine for coughs) with honey and give to your baby once a day. If the baby is 1-1½ years old then, you can give this quantity twice a day.
- Apply eucalyptus oil to baby's clothes, its pillow or bed or cot, as an aid to breath properly.
- Increase *haldi* (turmeric) in the *Balguti*.
- Apply oil heated with ajwain (caraway seeds) to the baby's back and chest. Next heat *kapoori pan/nagarvel* leaves (*Piper betle* or betel leaves) in a pan, making sure the temperature is bearable by the baby. Apply these warm leaves to the baby's chest and back, if there is congestion in its lungs. Re-heat the leaves whenever required, and continue the process for about 5 minutes.
- Boil milk with little *ajwain* (celery seed powder). Strain it and it can be given to the baby.

Umbilical Cord Infection/Swelling

In the womb, the umbilical cord connects the fetus to its mother. After birth, the cord is no longer needed. It is cut, and then clamped. The stump of the cord usually dries and falls off in a week or so. Sometimes, an umbilical cord infection causes the area under the stump to be inflamed, red and tender. The navel oozes a colored discharge and sometimes bleeds. Dried pus may be seen around the area.

- Wash navel with neem (Azadirachta indica) water and put a cotton ball dipped in neem oil onto the navel.
- You can sprinkle sandalwood powder on the navel.
- Frequently apply *lal chandan* (red sandalwood) to the navel. If you find it in powdered form, mix it with water and apply. If you have a stick of it, grind it on a stone with water and apply its paste.
- Heat castor oil with a paste of neem (Azadirachta indica) + *haldi* (turmeric), and apply this oil to the navel.

Loose Motions

- *Suthi* (dried ginger), *ativisa*, *nagarmotha* and kakadshingi should be ground with honey in *Balguti*
- It is important to watch out that the baby does not dehydrate, so add a pinch of salt + 1 teaspoon of *mistri* (crystalized sugar) to a cup of boiled water, and give 4-5 teaspoons of this to the baby at regular intervals.
- Add a few drops of lemon juice to milk and boil it. The milk will separate into a solid and a liquid. Strain the liquid + *mishri* (crystallized sugar) + lemon drops and give it to the baby, if the baby is a little older.

- If the above remedies do not work, please consult a doctor.
- Loose motions may also occur because of teething during months 7-18, so please treat it as a teething problem.

Teething

Generally, this problem doesn't arise if the baby is properly nourished and has a good level of calcium. Common problems associated with teething include loose motion, fever and vomiting.

- The baby may also have sore gums, so chewing *kharek* (dried dates) or *mulethi* (licorice) is good idea.
- Gently rub the gums of the baby with *amla* (Indian gooseberry) powder + honey.
- Gently massage gums with *til* (sesame) oil.
- Increase foods which are high in calcium, such as banana, yogurt, milk, *raagi*(finger millet) and cottage cheese.
- The homeopathic medicines *Calcarea Fluor* and *Calcarea Phosphorica* work very well too.

10.6   Baby's Milestones

Here is a list of the milestones your baby will reach and pass as time passes. Remember that each child grows in its own way, so your child may not meet all these milestones exactly as they are listed here – maturation can be more higgledy than that. However, in general you will find it very interesting to look out for these achievements, and celebrate them. They represent major steps in human development, and they all happen in the space of only a very few years.

1st Month

The baby will:

- sleep on her back and keep her legs folded.
- have a floppy head unless you support it, she has no control of her head.
- keep her fingers folded and make fist of them.
- look at the light and people.
- possibly turn towards family sounds, as her hearing is fully developed.

2nd Month

The baby will:

- gaze towards light and people.
- move its eyes from one side 180^0 across to the other side.
- try to suck its thumb.

3rd Month

The baby will:

- try to lift its head when sleeping on its abdomen, because now it has gain its head control.
- open its fist.
- play for some time with its toes and make sounds, like 'ghu ghour'.
- move its head in the direction of a voice.
- express joy, whenever you will call her. This means it now has a social smile.
- try to make small noises.

4th Month

The baby will:
- fully control its head, if you put it into a sitting position. Still this is not the right time to let it sit as its spine is not strong enough for sitting yet.
- play by tapping its legs on the floor, as the baby has now increased leg movement.
- try to cycle its legs.
- smile in the direction of a voice.
- try to watch moving things.

5th Month

The baby will:
- try to bring its leg towards its mouth, if you put the baby on its back.
- shrink paper and make a ball of it with finger movements, if you put paper in its hands.
- turn its face in the direction of a voice.
- start crying if the baby doesn't get an object it wants.

6th Month

The baby will:
- sit with support.
- hold things with its palms.
- indicate what it wants.
- recognize its mother better, and start crying upon seeing a stranger.
- start to move by itself.

7th Month

The baby will:
- try to turn onto its lateral side.
- start to learn chewing.
- tightly clench its lips, if you try to give a food it dislikes. This means the baby is now able to show its dislikes strongly, and also displays good muscle development.
- shift its weight about on its legs, if you hold the baby in a standing position.

8th Month

The baby will:
- start to sit without support.
- try to start crawling.
- Give response, if someone calls her.
- start to speak single letter words like "ma-ma", "da-da" and so on.

9th Month

The baby will:
- crawl better but only for short distances.
- try to stand up with support.
- sleep on its lateral side.
- start to throw things, and also express anger.

10th Month

The baby will:
- start to sit by itself.
- try to find its toys, which means the baby's memory has started to develop.
- try to walk with support.
- try to play with other kids of the same age, the start of being social.
- try to draw people's attention towards itself.
- hold the things with its fingers and thumb.

11th Month

The baby will:
- crawl smoothly for long distances.
- start to stand better, and will try to take small steps.
- put toys in the basket.
- say something like "no-no", if we try to take things from her.
- stand straight with very little support.

12th Month

The baby will:
- start walking.
- speak a few words like "mammy, moma, papa" and so on with understanding.
- recognize surrounding things.

1-1½ Years

The baby will:
- walk by itself.
- gives you a kiss if you ask for it.
- shows you the place where its shoes, socks, sandals and clothes are kept.
- climb steps by crawling up them.
- play the cup game and make a tower of 2 cups.
- drink water by itself with a cup.
- ask you to change its pants, if she peed in.
- start recognizing its body parts.
- starts following your instructions.
- identify common household objects like fan, light bulbs, chair etc.

1½-2 Years

The toddler will:

- run well.
- climb on furniture.
- try to put on shocks and shoes by itself.
- flip each page of a book.
- start to speak small sentences.

2½-3 Years

The toddler will:

- starts to hop.
- speaks well.

Around two years of age, your toddler might be able to use sentences of 2-3 words and say 'I', 'you' and 'me'. He'll learn and use lots of words, and will be easier to understand when she's talking.

At two and a half years of age, your toddler will be able to use sentences of 3-5 words, or even more. It'll start learning how to take turns when speaking, and might be able to have a short conversation with you. It'll start remembering what some things look like, for example that apples look red and round. It can probably wash its own hands, wash itself at bath time, feed itself, get dressed, although she's probably better at taking clothes off than putting them on! And she's still learning so you might still need to help.

3 to 4 Years

The child will:

- ride tricycle.
- speak well.
- wash its mouth, hands and legs by itself.
- do up her buttons.

10.7 Immunisation

Universal Immunisation Program

Age	Vaccines
Birth	BCG, OPV - 0
6 weeks	DPT – 1, OPV –1
10 weeks	DPT –2, OPV –2
14 weeks	DPT –3, OPV –3
9 months	Measles
16 -24 months	DPT booster, OPV - 4
5-6 years	DT*
10 years	TT**
16 years	TT
Pregnant women	TT (2 doses at 4 weeks interval)

....

So this now concludes the chapter about what is involved in caring for your baby … who turns miraculously into a toddler … who turns miraculously into a child!

The developmental progress towards full human maturity is just amazing, and it is happening at a phenomenal rate to someone who is so dear to you and your family. What you see happening in front of you in your child is one of the biggest intellectual steps that happens in a person's life.

And the things you learned about in this chapter will have helped you to support your child in this on-going development as healthily as possible.

With the aid of Ayurveda, you have given your child an absolutely wonderful start in life and helped it well on its way by now! Congratulations!

Postnatal Yoga

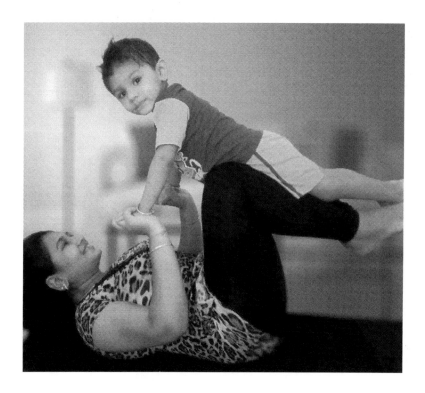

Motherhood is the most beautiful and a fulfilling phase in a woman's life. But sometimes it becomes tough when you have to deal with its after effects, such as weight gain, sagging of muscles, joint pain, backache, fatigue, hormonal imbalance, high blood pressure and weakness. Postnatal yoga is one of the best gift which you can give yourself to enjoy your motherhood at fullest.

Benefits of postnatal yoga

- Helps to reduce anxiety and depression
- Promotes stamina and strength
- Relieves stiffness and pains
- Strengthen pelvic floor muscles, abdominal and back
- Tones the abdominal muscles and helps to reduce extra fat
- Expands breathing and improves blood flow
- Promotes hormonal balance
- Promotes relaxation and deep rest
- Speeds up healing process
- Rejuvenates and recharges mind

Precautions before starting Postnatal Yoga

- Discuss with your doctor and ask for the right time to start practicing Yoga
- Do not drive yourself beyond limits. Always go gradually.
- Learn the yoga poses properly before practicing them on your own.
- If you have a vaginal delivery, you can start the following program as soon as you feel comfortable and a little charged up.
- If you had a c-section you can start following program after 6-8 weeks, this is general outline, so before you engage in yoga or any other exercise, ensure that you consult your doctor about your own health and wellbeing, to gauge your body's ability to undertake all kinds of physical stress, stretching and muscle pull.

11.1   Yoga for 1 – 8 week

This is the time for deep rest and relaxation but still you are allowed to walk around in the home after 15 days of your delivery but strenuous work must be restricted. It is advisable to adopt following light but very effective stretching to overcome pains and ache after delivery, generally the mother has to face.

1. Sukshma vyayam

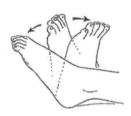

Ankle stretch

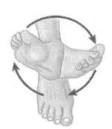

Ankle rotation

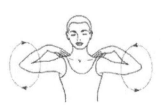

Shoulder rotation

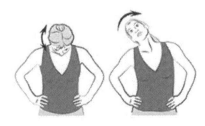

Neck rotation

2. Crocodile stretch 1

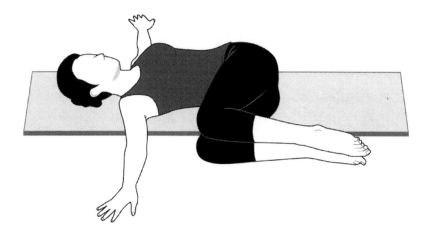

- Lie down on the floor with your hand spread on your shoulder level.
- Bend your both knees, feet together, touching to the hip.
- Slowly lower both your knees to your right side touching to the floor and move your face to your left side.
- Hold the stretch for 5 deep and slow breathing and then slowly come back. Repeat the same procedure with the next side
- Repeat for 3-5 rounds.

Benefits

- Works on the lower back. Generates good flexibility and flow in lower back and also removes pain if any.

3. Crocodile stretch 2

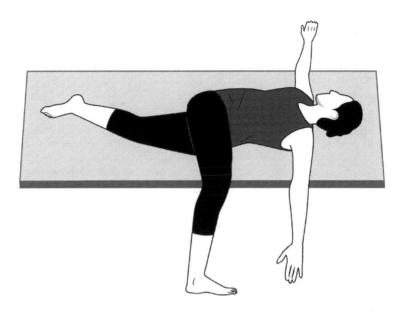

- Lie on your spine with hands spread to your shoulder level.
- Slowly lift your right leg at 90° and lower to your left side. Turn your face to your right.
- Hold the stretch for deep and slow 5 breathings and slowly come back. Repeat the same procedure with the next side.
- Repeat for 3-5 rounds.

Benefits

- Works on legs, hamstring and back muscles. Generates good flexibility and removes pains.

4. Crocodile stretch 3

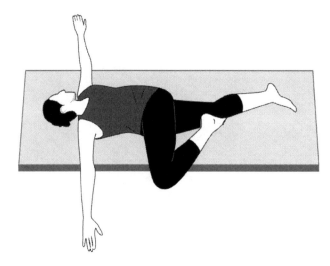

- Lie down straight on the floor with hands spread to your shoulder level.
- Bend your right knee and place your right foot on your left knee.
- Slowly lower your right knee to your left side possibly touching the floor and move your face to your right side.
- Hold this stretch for deep and slow 5 breathings and slowly come back. Repeat the same procedure with the next side.
- Repeat for 3-5 rounds.

Benefits

- Removes back pain and gives strength.

5. Crocodile stretch 4

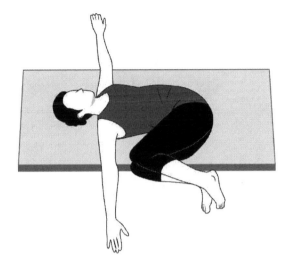

- Take a supine position on the floor with hands spread to your shoulder level.
- Bend both your knees and bring towards your chest.
- Slowly lower your both knees to your right side and move your face to your left.
- Hold the posture for deep and slow 5 breathings. Inhale and come back to the center and repeat the process to the next side.
- Repeat for 3-5 rounds.

Benefits

- Removes pain and discomfort of the middle back.

6. Modify hamstring stretch

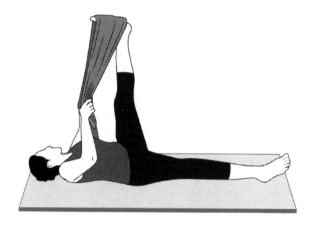

- Take a supine position on the floor. Hold a towel or scarf in your hands.
- Lift your right leg, bend your knee and loop the towel around your right sole and straighten your leg at 90°. Hold the stretch for 30 seconds and slowly lower your leg.
- Repeat the same procedure with your next leg.
- Same stretch also can be taken in sitting position.

Benefits

- Stretches your back and hamstring muscles and easies the pain if any.

7. Hip lift

- Check figure 3, in Ch-3 – 'Prenatal Yoga' for instructions.
- Repeat the procedure for 10 rounds.

8. Cat Cow posture

- Check figure 5, in Ch-3 – 'Prenatal Yoga' for instructions.
- Repeat the procedure for 10 rounds

9. Cat cow with belly rotation

- Check figure 16, in Ch-3 – 'Prenatal Yoga' for instructions.
- Repeat the procedure for 15 rounds

10. Kegel Exercise (Ashwini mudra)

- Check figure 8, in Ch-3 – 'Prenatal Yoga' for instructions.
- Repeat the procedure for 30 rounds

11. Belly Rotation

- Check figure 11, in Ch-3 – 'Prenatal Yoga' for instructions.
- Repeat the procedure for 10 rounds

12. Anulom Vilom Pranayama

- Check in Ch-3 – 'Prenatal Yoga' for instructions.
- Practice Pranayama for 10 minutes.

13. Om Chanting

Repeat for 10 rounds.

11.2 Yoga for 9 – 16 week

This is the time to gradually start with some easy but very effective exercise to prepare your body for a full yoga session after 15 weeks. You should continue the above mentioned stretching and gradually start below mentioned exercises simultaneously.

1. Leg raising

- Check figure 2, in Ch-3 – 'Prenatal Yoga' for instructions.
- Start with 10 counts with each leg and gradually increase it up to 20 counts.

2. Leg rotation

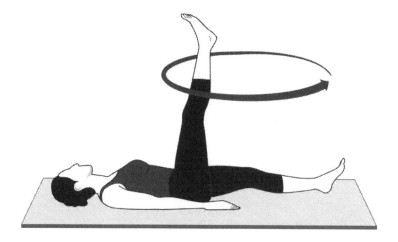

- Lie down straight on your back with hands near to your body.
- Lift your right leg and make big circles without bending your knee.
- Gradually increase the circles from 5 to 15 counts, clock and anticlock wise each.
- Repeat the same process with your next leg.

Benefits

- Helps to reduce abdominal fat and tones up thigh muscles

3. Cycling

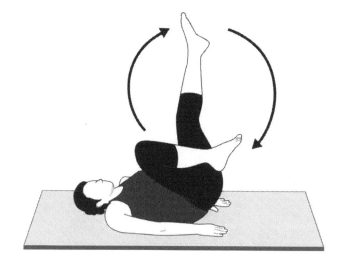

- Lie down on the floor with your hands near to your body.
- Slowly move your legs like cycling.
- Gradually increase the count from 20 to 50 cycles clockwise and then anti-clockwise.

Benefits

- Reduces fat from the abdomen and thighs.
- Strengthens pelvic and lower back muscle

4. Both legs cycling

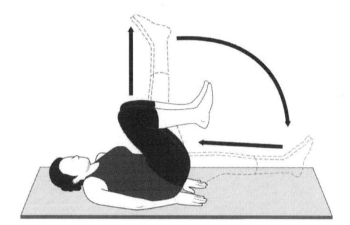

- Lie down straight on your back with your hands under your hips, for supporting your back and hips.
- Slowly moves both your legs in a cycling motion.
- Make sure that your hands give proper support to your back so that you don't hurt your back while cycling.
- Gradually increase the count from 7 to 20 cycles clockwise and then anticlock-wise. Be gentle with your body.

Benefits

- Excellent workout for your abdominal muscles.

5. Both leg raising

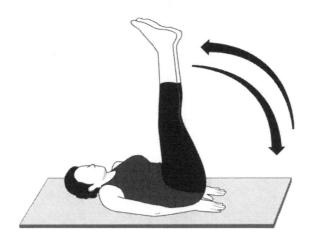

- Lie down straight on your back with your hands under your hips, to support your back and hips.
- Slowly lift your both legs at 90°, keeping your knees straight. Then slowly go down without a jerk.
- Repeat the procedure for 5 to 15 counts.

Benefits

- Reduces excess fat and tones the abdominal muscles.

6. Both leg rotations

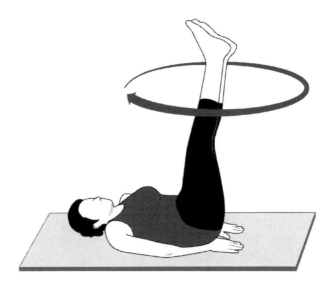

- Lie down straight on your back with your hands under your hips.
- Slowly rotate both your legs to make big circles. Make sure to keep your knees straight.
- Gradually increase the counts from 5 to 12, clock and anticlockwise.

Benefits

- Reduces tummy fat, tones and flattens it.

7. Kapalbhati Pranayam

- Sit in a comfortable position where your spine is straight and your abdomen is not compressed. One can sit in Padmasana, Sukhasana or Vajrasana.
- Bring your awareness to your lower belly.
- Inhale through both nostrils deeply.
- Contract your low belly, forcing out the breath in a short burst.
- As you quickly release the contraction, your inhalation should be automatic and passive- your focus should be on exhaling.
- Begin slowly, aiming for 65-70 contractions per minute. Gradually quicken the pace, aiming for 95-105 contractions per minute. Always go at your own pace and take a break in between whenever feel like.
- Start practice for 3-5 minutes and gradually increase up to 10 minutes.

11.3   From the 16 week onwards

- Now you are ready for full yoga sessions.
- One can also practice Suryanamskar, Uttanpadasan, Pavanmuktasan, Naukasana, Sarvangasan, Halasana, Bhujangasan, Dhanurasan, Butterfly, Paschimotanasan, Uddiyan Bandha etc.

....

Miscellaneous

12.1 Average Height & Weight chart of Baby

HEIGHT / WEIGHT CHART

Average height and weight of boys at different ages

Age	Weight (kg)	Height (cm)
Birth	3.3	50.5
3 months	6.0	61.1
6 months	7.8	67.8
9 months	9.2	72.3
1 year	10.2	76.1
2 years	12.3	85.6
3 years	14.6	94.9
4 years	16.7	102.9
5 years	18.7	109.9
6 years	20.7	116.1
7 years	22.9	121.7
8 years	25.3	127.0
9 years	28.1	132.2
10 years	31.4	137.5

Average height and weight of girls at different ages

Age	Weight (kg)	Height (cm)
Birth	3.2	49.9
3 months	5.4	60.2
6 months	7.2	66.6
9 months	8.6	71.1
1 year	9.5	75.0
2 years	11.8	84.5
3 years	14.1	93.9
4 years	16.0	101.6
5 years	17.7	108.4
6 years	19.5	114.6
7 years	21.8	120.6
8 years	24.8	126.4
9 years	28.5	132.2
10 years	32.5	138.3

12.2   Teething Chart

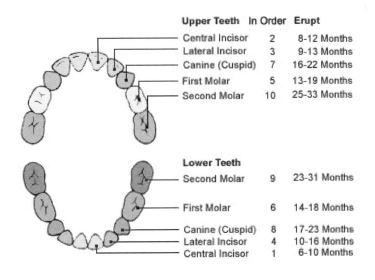

Upper Teeth	In Order	Erupt
Central Incisor	2	8-12 Months
Lateral Incisor	3	9-13 Months
Canine (Cuspid)	7	16-22 Months
First Molar	5	13-19 Months
Second Molar	10	25-33 Months

Lower Teeth		
Second Molar	9	23-31 Months
First Molar	6	14-18 Months
Canine (Cuspid)	8	17-23 Months
Lateral Incisor	4	10-16 Months
Central Incisor	1	6-10 Months

12.3 Estimated Date of Delivery

Your Estimated Date of Delivery Chart

January	1	2	3	4	5	6	7	8	9	10	11	12	13	14	15	16	17	18	19	20	21	22	23	24	25	26	27	28	29	30	31
October	8	9	10	11	12	13	14	15	16	17	18	19	20	21	22	23	24	25	26	27	28	29	30	31	1/Nov	2/Nov	3/Nov	4/Nov	5/Nov	6/Nov	7/Nov

February	1	2	3	4	5	6	7	8	9	10	11	12	13	14	15	16	17	18	19	20	21	22	23	24	25	26	27	28
November	8	9	10	11	12	13	14	15	16	17	18	19	20	21	22	23	24	25	26	27	28	29	30	1/Dec	2/Dec	3/Dec	4/Dec	5/Dec

March	1	2	3	4	5	6	7	8	9	10	11	12	13	14	15	16	17	18	19	20	21	22	23	24	25	26	27	28	29	30	31
December	6	7	8	9	10	11	12	13	14	15	16	17	18	19	20	21	22	23	24	25	26	27	28	29	30	31	1/Jan	2/Jan	3/Jan	4/Jan	5/Jan

April	1	2	3	4	5	6	7	8	9	10	11	12	13	14	15	16	17	18	19	20	21	22	23	24	25	26	27	28	29	30
January	6	7	8	9	10	11	12	13	14	15	16	17	18	19	20	21	22	23	24	25	26	27	28	29	30	31	1/Feb	2/Feb	3/Feb	4/Feb

May	1	2	3	4	5	6	7	8	9	10	11	12	13	14	15	16	17	18	19	20	21	22	23	24	25	26	27	28	29	30	31
February	5	6	7	8	9	10	11	12	13	14	15	16	17	18	19	20	21	22	23	24	25	26	27	28	1/Mar	2/Mar	3/Mar	4/Mar	5/Mar	6/Mar	7/Mar

June	1	2	3	4	5	6	7	8	9	10	11	12	13	14	15	16	17	18	19	20	21	22	23	24	25	26	27	28	29	30
March	8	9	10	11	12	13	14	15	16	17	18	19	20	21	22	23	24	25	26	27	28	29	30	31	1/Apr	2/Apr	3/Apr	4/Apr	5/Apr	6/Apr

July	1	2	3	4	5	6	7	8	9	10	11	12	13	14	15	16	17	18	19	20	21	22	23	24	25	26	27	28	29	30	31
April	7	8	9	10	11	12	13	14	15	16	17	18	19	20	21	22	23	24	25	26	27	28	29	30	1/May	2/May	3/May	4/May	5/May	6/May	7/May

August	1	2	3	4	5	6	7	8	9	10	11	12	13	14	15	16	17	18	19	20	21	22	23	24	25	26	27	28	29	30	31
May	8	9	10	11	12	13	14	15	16	17	18	19	20	21	22	23	24	25	26	27	28	29	30	31	1/Jun	2/Jun	3/Jun	4/Jun	5/Jun	6/Jun	7/Jun

September	1	2	3	4	5	6	7	8	9	10	11	12	13	14	15	16	17	18	19	20	21	22	23	24	25	26	27	28	29	30
June	8	9	10	11	12	13	14	15	16	17	18	19	20	21	22	23	24	25	26	27	28	29	30	1/Jul	2/Jul	3/Jul	4/Jul	5/Jul	6/Jul	7/Jul

October	1	2	3	4	5	6	7	8	9	10	11	12	13	14	15	16	17	18	19	20	21	22	23	24	25	26	27	28	29	30	31
July	8	9	10	11	12	13	14	15	16	17	18	19	20	21	22	23	24	25	26	27	28	29	30	31	1/Aug	2/Aug	3/Aug	4/Aug	5/Aug	6/Aug	7/Aug

November	1	2	3	4	5	6	7	8	9	10	11	12	13	14	15	16	17	18	19	20	21	22	23	24	25	26	27	28	29	30
August	8	9	10	11	12	13	14	15	16	17	18	19	20	21	22	23	24	25	26	27	28	29	30	31	1/Sep	2/Sep	3/Sep	4/Sep	5/Sep	6/Sep

December	1	2	3	4	5	6	7	8	9	10	11	12	13	14	15	16	17	18	19	20	21	22	23	24	25	26	27	28	29	30	31
September	7	8	9	10	11	12	13	14	15	16	17	18	19	20	21	22	23	24	25	26	27	28	29	30	1/Oct	2/Oct	3/Oct	4/Oct	5/Oct	6/Oct	7/Oct

Instruction for the use of the above table

Find the date of your last menstrual period in the first row. The date shown below this is the EDD (expected date of delivery.). The actual date could be within the span of eight days on either side of the EDD. According to Ayurvedic literature, the duration of pregnancy is nine months and nine days. Counted in this manner, the EDD falls four to five days before that acquired from the table.

Example: If your last menstrual period is January 1 then the due date is October 8, +/- 8 days, indicating anytime between 1 to 15 October.

12.4 RECIPES

1. Suthi Ladoo (Ginger ball)

Suthi ladoo is a very traditional recipe in India which is given to the mother after delivery. Suthi works excellently in the postnatal period as it aids digestion, purifies the uterus, pacifies vata and also prevent from backache.

Ingredients:

Suthi (dry ginger powder) powder: 20g.
Pure Ghee: 40gm approx
Grated jaggery: 40gm

Add jaggery to the suthi powder and mix well. Add the liquid ghee to the above mixture and make small balls in the size of grapes. Store in an airtight container. It is good to have one ladoo every morning on an empty stomach.

2. Raab:

This is one more Indian traditional recipe which is very important in postnatal period.

Ingredients:

Wheat flour 2 tsp
Ghee 2 tbsp approx
Water 1 glass
Jaggery as per test

Suthi ½ tsp
Piplimool powder ½ tsp
Grated dry coconut 1 tsp

Take ghee in a pan, keep the flame low, add wheat flour in it and stir till it turns pinkish, then add water and jaggery, stir till jaggery dissolves completely. After that add suthi, piplimool and grated dry coconut. Your raab is ready & have it hot. Said quantity will prepare almost a big bowl, it is good to have this much quantity in the morning after suthi ladoo.

One can even use Bajari (millet flour) instead of wheat flour.

3. Methi Ladoo:

Methi has lots of benefits like it enhance breast milk production, help to lose weight, aid digestion and also prevent from joint pain.

Ingredients:

Methi seed (fenugreek seeds): 50gm   Almond powder: 50gm
Piplimool powder: 50gm   Wheat flour: 10 gm
Dry grated coconut: 50gh   Jaggery: 400 -500 gm as per test
Eatable Gum: 50gm   Ghee: 300 gm
Raisins (kismis): 50gm
Suthi powder: 75gm

1. Take a pan. Dry roast the wheat flour over a slow flame while stirring continuously till it turns golden brown. Keep it aside.
2. Grind methi seed in fine powder and roast it in the same way as above, keep aside.
3. Now add ¼ (of total quantity) ghee to the pan and add gum in it & roast till the spluttering stops.
4. Now add wheat flour, methi powder , dry coconut, raisins in pan and mix well then turn off flame
5. Now take another pan add remaining ghee and heat it, then add jaggery to it, stir well until it appears in nice liquid form of golden color.
6. Now add wheat flour mixture and suthi powder, piplimool powder, almond powder and mix well, turn off flame.
7. Now make round ladoos of the mixture and store in an airtight container.

4. Eatable Gum Ladoo (Gond):

After pregnancy, this Ladoo is good for nursing mother as it increases the breast milk for the baby and helps the mother's body to recover fast. It also strengthens the back bone.

Ingredients:

Dry coconut powder 100 gm
Dry kharik powder 100 gm
Dink (Gum) 50 gms
Almonds 50 gms
Pista 50 gms
Cashew nuts 50 gms
Kismis 50 gms
Roasted poppy seeds (khus khus) 1 tbsp
Ghee 1 cup
Cardamom powder 1 tsp
For Syrup: Sugar 2 cup + milk 1/2 cup

1. Take thick bottom pan, heat 1 tbsp ghee, and dry roast kharik powder for 3-4 min on low flame. Repeat the procedure for coconut, almond, pista, cashew nuts keep it aside.
2. In pan heat 1/2 cup ghee and fry dink. Take out dink, crush them lightly with hand and keep it aside.
3. Now in the blender make coarse powder of almond and pista. Keep it aside.
4. Now in mixing bowl, mix all ingredients kharik powder, coconut powder, coarse powder of almond pista, kismis, cashew nuts, roasted poppy seeds, cardamom powder. Keep it aside.

Now make sugar syrup. For that put the milk and sugar in a thick bottom pan and bring to a boil keeping medium-high flame. When the syrup comes to a boil, turn the heat down to medium and stir to dissolve the sugar completely. . Pour the above mixture in syrup and mix well once it turns in thick solid mixture & turn off the flame. Take a spoonful of mixture in hand and make ladoos.

5. Bhaidku:

This is very nutritive preparation and also very soft for the digestive system. One can have this preparation at dinner time as there are less options for variety in dinner in the first 45 days of delivery.

Ingredients:

Green Mung dal: ½ cup	Water
Bajri (millet): 2 cup	Salt as per taste
Rice: ½ cup	Black pepper
Wheat: ½ cup	Suthi
Ghee	Turmeric powder

1. Take green mung dal, bajri, rice, wheat together and grind it in flour.
2. Take a pan, put 4-5 tsp of ghee add ½ cup of above mixed flour and roast it in low flame till it turns pinkish.
3. Now add 2 cup of water to it, stir properly then add salt, suthi, black pepper, turmeric powder as per taste.
4. The mixture will create a thick pest, turn off flame and have it hot.

6. Kheer:

This is a nice sweet dish, with cooling nature for the body. Very good to consume during pregnancy as it increases Oja & Bala (strength).

Ingredients:

Full cream milk: 5 cup
Rice (washed): ¼ cup
Sugar: ½ cup
Raisins: 10-15
Almond (blanched): 4-5

1. Boil the rice and milk in a deep pan.
2. Simmer over low flame, stirring occasionally till the rice is cooked and the milk becomes thick.
3. When done add sugar, raisins and almond
4. Stir till sugar gets dissolved properly. Transfer into a serving dish and garnish with almonds.
5. Serve hot or chilled.

Instead of rice one can even use semolina (rava) and make semolina Kheer. This recipe is very good for mother during pregnancy and also good for the baby at the age of 7-8 month plus.

7. Sheera:

Again this is very traditional recipe of India and widely use after delivery. This recipe nourishes the mother's body & brings good energy & strength.

Ingredients:

Water – 1 ¼ cup
Ghee – ¼ cup
Fine sooji or rava or semolina – ½ cup
White granulated sugar – ½ cup
cardamom powder – ¼ teaspoon
Almonds, cashews, and raisins – 2 tablespoons, chopped

1) Take ghee and fine semolina in a pan. Turn the heat on low-medium.

2) Start roasting the sooji with stirring constantly.

3) While ghee is melting, take water in a saucepan on another stove. Turn the heat on medium. Let it come to a simmer.

4) Back to the roasting sooji, ghee is melted. Do stir constantly with spatula.

5) Keep stirring and roasting until it gets a slight brown color till you get the nice toasty aroma of sooji. You will notice that ghee is oozing out and it starts to bubble. It took me 7-8 minutes.

6) Now add warm water slowly. Be very careful, it will get very bubbly and will splutter a lot so immediately mix it. Cook with stirring continuously till water is absorbed. This will be done very quickly, about in 2 minutes.

7) Now add sugar, Mix well until sugar melts.

8) Lastly add cardamom powder, chopped cashews and almonds and raisins (if using).

9) Sheera or halwa is ready to serve. You can just spoon it in a bowl. Or go fancy. Tightly pack sheera in a katori or designed bowl, remove it to a plate upside down. Do this while sheera is hot or warm to get smooth surface.

This is very nice recipe for the mother and also for the baby 7-8 months plus. One can also use wheat flour instead of Suji and remaining procedure is the same. Mother should have it hot and it can be given at room temperature to the baby. Instead of sugar one can use jaggery as a better option if you like.

8. Katlu (Saubhagya Suthi pakka)

Katlu is a mixture of a lot of different ayurvedic herbs mixed together. Katlu is given to new mother to help her recover. Katlu powder is readily available in the market. It is good for new mother to have it in the morning. This is an excellent recipe to increase breast milk and give strength to the mother.

Ingredients:

Ghee 1 tbsp
Jaggery 2 tsp
Katlu powder 3 tsp

Heat ghee in a pan, then add jaggery. Stir constantly until it turns in light brown. Now add katlu powder to it and mix well. Your katlu is ready, serve hot.

Herbs in katlu powder:

- Asedio
- Aasan
- Baldana
- Bedaana
- Chavak
- Chimed
- Chopchini
- Ekhro
- Gokhru
- Kamalkakadi
- Kamarkas
- Kavachaa
- Laalbaman
- Laving
- Mari
- Moglai
- Narguda
- Peepar
- Piplimool
- Saalam
- Safed Bamag
- Safed Mari
- Safed Musli
- Satavari
- Suthi
- Surijan
- Tavkeer
- Tejfal
- Taj
- Variyali
- Vekario
- Cheetrak

Scientific names of medicinal plants

Aerand (castor)	Ricinus communis L.
Aserio	Common cress
Ashwagandha	Withania Somnifera
Ativisa	Aconitum heterophyllum
Bhojpatra	Betula utilis D.
Brahmi	Bacopa monnieri
Gokshur	Tribulus terrestris
Guggal	commiphora mukul
Harde	Terminalia chebula
Hira bol	Commiphora myrrha
Indrajav	Holarrhena pubescens
Jivanti	Leptadenia reticulata
Kadiatu	Andrographis paniculata
Kakach	Pongamia glabra vent
Kakadshingi	Rhus succedanea
Kamal kakadi	Lotus seed
Malkangari	Celastrus paniculatus
Nagarmotha	Cyperus rotundus
Nagkeshar	Mesua ferrea
Piplimool	Long pepper Root
Shatavari	Asparagus racemosus
Suganthi Vado	Vetiveria Zizanioides
Tej bal	Toothache tree
Vaidari	Ipomoea digitata
Vaja	Acorus calamus L.
Vakumba	Careya arborea rox B.
Vavding	Embelia ribes
Yestimadhu	Glycyrrhiza glabra

Glossary

Apana vayu	Apana vayu is one of the types of vata, which is most active in the pelvis and lower abdomen, governs the eliminative functions (excretion, urination, menstruation) and the downward and outward flow of energy in the body. There is lots of importance to balance apana vayu for ideal labor.
dosha	Vata, pitta and Kapha- The three major fundctioning forces in the human body. When one or more of these 'doshas' is out of equilibrium, it brings disease. The root of all discomforts can be

	traced back to the imbalance of the doshas.
Guna	Good Values
kapha	kapha governs the structure of the body. It is the principle that holds the cells together and forms the muscle, fat, bone, and sinew.
Ojas	Life force energy
pitta	Pitta governs all heat, metabolism and transformation in the mind and body.
satsang	a spiritual discourse
sattvik	The Sattvic diet is said to restore and maintain a sattvik or sentient state of living. Nuts, Veggies, Dairy, Whole grain, Fruits, pulses etc.
Shukra dhatu	Male semen or female egg
vata	Vata governs all movement in the mind and body. It controls blood flow, elimination of wastes, breathing and the movement of thoughts across the mind.

Reference Books

- Charak Samhita
- Charak sharirshthan
- Sushrut Samhita
- Sushrut sharirshthan
- Ashtangasangraha
- Hatha yoga pradipika
- Ayurvedic Grbha Sanskar
- Tandurashti tamara hathma
- Putrada ane Parnu
- Baa ane Badak
- Gherand shamhita
- Grey's anatomy

Made in the USA
Columbia, SC
15 November 2022

71313449R00113